An en

MW01247424

DRUG ADDICTION

Substance - Abuse, Alcohol Addiction

Practical Guidelines for Success Oriented,
De-addiction and Rehabilitation

Perseverance
By
The Victim~ Medical Faculty = Family

Dr (Mrs) Saroje Sanan

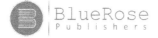

BlueRose
Publishers

First Published in August 2020

ISBN: 978-81-947240-0-1

BLUEROSE PUBLISHERS
www.bluerosepublishers.com
info@bluerosepublishers.com
+91 8882 898 898

Cover Design:
Mohd Arif

Typographic Design:
Ayushi Garg

Distributed by: BlueRose, Amazon, Flipkart, Shopclues

FOREWORD

In 1993-1994, during the term of my husband Sh. Karan Bir Singh Sidhu, IAS as DC, Amritsar, the "Deaddiction cum Rehabilitation Centre" was setup under the aegis of the District Branch of the Indian Red Cross Society.

Dr. (Mrs.) Saroje Sanan, MBBS(DLH), Ph.D(EDIN), M.N.A.M.S.(INDIA) and Dr. J.P.S. Bhatia, MD Psychiatrist were responsible for operationalizing and enabling the functioning of the Centre.

Many others, carefully acknowledged by Dr.(Mrs.) Saroje Sanan, contributed their valuable services and donations, and many a life was saved due to their diligence and compassionate medical care.

It therefore gives me great pleasure to write the foreword to this compilation, which discuses various aspects of the disease 'addiction'.

Dr. Sanan's knowledge and experience in the management of the "Deaddiction cum Rehabilitation Centre" at Amritsar is a very valuable contribution to those engaged in tackling the menace of addiction currently a focus for Punjab.

I wish her the very best in taking her message far and wide and especially to all who need it, in this critical area of care, impacting our generations to come.

"With best wishes"

Poonam Khaira Sidhu, IRS
Life Member
Indian Red Cross and Hospital Welfare Section

Dated: 09.08.2019

Perceptions and Sentiments --- Of The Author

This compilation on drug-addiction / substance abuse / alcohol addiction and its management / treatment is dedicated to the memory of those "unfortunate victims" who lost their precious lives at the altar of this terrible disease — this menace continues to be an enigmatic social and medical challenge.

"They" walked on this road on their own, which led them to their own ruin.

The families remained unaware of the "fatal" journey of their loved ones.

The 'custodians' of their lives could not prevent "it".

All failed to contribute to the " maximum " to save them.

"They" knew not, the rest know not enough. Loss of precious lives continues.

The victims of Drug-addiction/Substance- abuse and alcoholism are considered a stigma by most and they are rejected by the family and friends.

The contents of the different chapters is an effort towards a more complete understanding of the disease of Drug/Substance-abuse / Alcohol and its victims, and their families. This disease has devoured thousands of precious young lives and the disaster continues unabated and has assumed awesome magnitude by now.

Contd....

The efforts, to contain this menace are obvious but have not proven enough, because important aspects are neither fully recognised nor attended to.

Re-Assessment of the planned Medical Care and existing Rehabilitation efforts so far is the call of the hour.

Author :-

Dr. (Mrs.) Saroje Sanan. M.B.B.S. (Dlh) , Ph.D. (Edin), M.N.A.M.S. (India).

Former professor and Head of the Department Of Pharmacology, Government Medical College Amritsar. Former President , Indian Pharmacological Society Amritsar. Former Project Director, The Red Cross De-addiction-cum-Rehabilitation Centre. The Indian Red Cross Society District Branch Amritsar (From 1995-2010/11) initially as project co-ordinator / project-in-charge-cum administrator.

My Gratitude To......

I am grateful to GOD —the omnipotent, for giving me the opportunity to work in The Red Cross De-addiction-cum-Rehabilitation Centre (R.C.D.A.R.C), Amritsar. This opportunity gave my life a new direction, a new purpose of living for others; it also helped me to understand the significance of this change in the priorities of my life.

An unseen power had taken hold of my thoughts; these became increasingly centred on the care of the drug-addicts admitted in The Red Cross De-addiction-cum-Rehab. Centre (R.C.D.A.R.C.), Amritsar, to the exclusion of all my other life routines. Each successive day infused me with increased concern for the addicts under treatment and the zeal and the capacity to work tirelessly, overcoming purposeless personal interests and routines of my earlier life.

In 2003, my dependence on a walking aid due to osteoarthritis of the hip joints came as a blessing in disguise. Walking was not only difficult but also very painful and, an experience of a very brief period of deep emotional hurt. *The almighty who had designed it for me, also helped me to understand his message for my life , henceforth.*

It is my unshakable belief that this disguised blessing was for my inner progress and for a more meaningful contribution to the work assigned by

Him. He also blessed me with enough physical endurance, perseverance and patience to understand the drug-addicts and their woes and also of their families and work tirelessly day after day.

Dr. J. P. S. Bhatia, a qualified and expert psychiatrist was the Dr. in-charge of R.C.D.A.R.C. Amritsar, and this too was a God-ordained gift to the Centre, he contributed his dedicated care of the Drug-users from his first day in the Centre in 1995 to the last day of its functioning in the year 2011. I learnt a great deal from him and so did the other staff members who were motivated to give their best. The Red Cross Office extended unstinted support under all circumstances.

By God's grace successive Patrons and Chair Persons of The Red Cross De-addiction cum Rehabilitation Centre Amritsar were a source of helpful encouragement all through the years that the Centre functioned.

A Contemplative Compilation of Woeful Arduous Life Journey of a Drug-Addict And His Family And His Redeemers

(Compilation in the form of a Book by the author is based on her observations and applicable management conclusions as Project In-charge in The Red Cross De-addiction/De-addiction-cum-Rehabilitation Centre, Amritsar, Punjab).

The problem of drug-addiction demands focus on initiating factors and promoting influences, its acceptance as a disease and its salient features, timely detection and initiation of treatment. Additionally an ideal role of the De-addiction Centres and the Doctor in-charge.

The Distinctive Features of the Compilation include

Acceptance of Drug-Addiction as a disease, understanding each victim in-depth, early detection and consultation for indoor treatment. Individual-specific, situation-specific and an EMPATHIC approach during Indoor treatment in a De-addiction/De-addiction-cum-Rehabilitation Centre. Family support through all the above stages followed by after-care precautions at home and prolonged follow-up for sustained recovery, rehabilitation and drug-free life.

This Book is an effort towards a dispassionate analysis of our successes and failures of the De-addiction treatment regimes planned for reducing the awesome increase in the addicted population.

Dispassionate analysis of success and short comings in minimizing / solving the De-addiction menace is discussed in the chapter that follows.

Well-meaning steps over the past many years by the State Administration, NGOs, social organisations and individual social workers are commendable efforts for public awareness and treatment of the addicts.

The present scenario of addiction beckons us to make a dispassionate analysis of these efforts in the face of a galloping increase in the prevailing addiction menace engulfing in its fold all age groups irrespective of social and financial status.

The young population of the state/country, the real strength of rising India, are becoming crumbling pillars of the society.

AN ATTEMPT TOWARDS A DISPASSIONATE ANALYSIS .....

We have to accept an undeniable fact that years have rolled by and we are still moving by inches towards an elusive success in solving the problem of drug addiction menace (re-assessment of the ongoing efforts and considerations of the necessary measures).

Drug-addiction menace is increasing at an awesome pace and engulfing in its fold the old and young alike irrespective of social and financial status. The most alarming aspect is that the young population of the state/country, expected to be the strength of rising India, are becoming crumbling pillars of the society because this age group is increasingly becoming the victim of Drug-abuse.

I have been following the daily news pertaining to the seizures of addictive substances, opium, heroin, smack, intoxicating tablets etc. That this menace has invaded the teaching institutions and the fact that there is a gradual lowering of age group of those who are using the addictive substances,is a very alarming aspect of the problem. **Alongside this disheartening picture there is also news on daily basis, of the commendable efforts of State Administration, NGOs, Social Organisations and Individual Social Workers, who all are contributing towards limiting the addiction menace by various individual and collective efforts.**

The present scenario of addiction menace beckons us to make a dispassionate analysis of all the well-meaning efforts enumerated above, so that we make these more effective and result oriented. I feel that I will be failing in my responsibility towards the cause of Drug / Substance –abuse menace if I do not draw the attention of all well-wishers to a very pertinent question that remains unanswered as to why the number of drug/substance abuse victims has been on increase all these years, in spite of well-intentioned measures by all.

- Where are we failing in our approach to the problem? Is it in terms of knowledge, methodology of de-addiction regimes or sincerity of purpose in our attempts . The addicted population has been increasing unabated.

- The targeted success has eluded all of us (the State efforts, efforts of N.G.Os, private organisations and the treatment efforts by the Medical Faculty) in spite of all the well-intentioned programmes attempted through various means, year after year.

- It is a very valid question as to where and how we have failed or are failing in our efforts to reduce the 'addicted population' successfully. We must seek an answer to this question.

- It is high time that we analyse and bring to the forefront the important causes without being judgemental and indulging in blame games and without criticism and condemnation; only a truthful analysis is required to arrive at some constructive conclusions. This should be followed by a concentrated and consecrated approach for integral and effective planning to deal with the awesome problem of the unchecked spread of drug addiction.

- For each one of us who feels concerned for the welfare of the addicts, it is a moment of a genuine search for the truth of the present situation in order to apply a more successful approach.

   A focused analysis of the measures/steps that have been taken over all these years to manage Drug addiction problem, is required. A dispassionate assessment of the utility of these is warranted.

   After much contemplation and hesitation, I have decided to comment on this delicate subject. If I do not do so I would be failing in my responsibility towards this cause of increasing

Drug-addiction menace. One must assess truthfully the preventive and curative steps taken to manage addiction menace overall these years. It seems we are fighting a losing battle.

• So far the generally attributed causes considered responsible for the continuous increase of addicted population are as follows: (a) Easy availability of the addictive substances. (b) Lack of awareness about increasing drug-addiction menace in the public. (c) Poor employment opportunities for the young.

The possible role of inadequate and incomplete de-addiction regimes, as a cause of vulnerability to relapses, is not appreciated to the extent that it should have been. Relapses play a substantial role in the increase of addiction menace and this deserves serious consideration.

During my tenure of managing the Red Cross De-addiction cum Rehabilitation Centre (R.C.D.A.R.C.), Amritsar, Punjab, from year 1995-2010/11 , initially as Project Co-ordinator and finally as Project Director-cum-Administrator. I interacted with each new patient to understand him and learn about his 'Disease' of Drug-addiction/Substance-abuse/ Alcohol addiction. Fifteen years gave me long enough opportunity to look after them, know them and their 'Disease'.

Every addict was my teacher and I learnt from him. The addicts shared their stories, their sentiments and also coherent thoughts during their lucid moments. This helped me to analyse the causes of limited success in the treatment of addiction. The most apparent cause was the occurrence of relapses and the relapsed cases added substantially to the addicted population. **Relapses occur due to short duration of indoor/in-house de-addiction treatment and poor follow-up and after care.**

The Ministry of Social Justice and Empowerment M.S.J.E. New Delhi , recommends a minimum period of one-month Indoor/In-house De-addiction treatment. These recommendations were followed in The Red Cross De-addiction-cum-Rehabilitation Centre, Amritsar, Punjab.

Duration of Indoor/ In-house De-addiction treatment in the Centres is an important key factor which influences Recovery and Rehabilitation of the Addict

Any De-addiction-cum-Rehabilitation Centre providing only fifteen days indoor treatment is not justifiable and De-addiction regime of this nature becomes a misnomer. This is as much applicable to The De-addiction Camps held for short duration from time to time for De-addiction treatment.

The short duration of Indoor treatment (ten to fifteen days only) detoxifies but does not de-addict the individual and the treated addict remains vulnerable to relapses. The phase of De-addiction starts after the initial phase of detoxification; the detoxified addict becomes more responsive to counselling and gradually moves towards self-realisation of the value of becoming drug-free.(The details are given in Chapter – 2 Pg 11 and sub-chapter – 6 on Pg 33)

In the interest of managing the present magnitude of addiction menace, I feel it is my moral responsibility to give my opinion; justifying it on the basis of my own experience during the management of

R.C.D.A.R.C. Amritsar for a continuous period of fifteen years, and this is the basis of my comments.

The addicts suffering from The Disease of Drug-addiction have to be given special care, intensive in approach, with selfless dedication and devotion and almost inexhaustible patience and continuity of goodwill, in spite of the provocative behaviour and mood swings of the addicts periodically, during their stay in the Centre.

Serving in R.C.D.A.R.C. Amritsar was a long enough opportunity to understand their thoughts and feelings and develop an emotional bond with them. I learnt all lessons while interacting with almost each admitted addict day after day, accepting them affectionately in-spite of their aggressive behavioural outbursts.

'The unquestionable dictum' for their welfare is to know the addict as an individual, his disease of drug-addiction , have an **empathic approach** and follow the principle of individual-specific and situation-specific management while they are under treatment.

- Addicts rewarded our efforts in R.C.D.A.R.C and our compassionate approach. This gave them the confidence to share their sentiments and thoughts with us. This was our reward.

- Our tenacity and our capacity to carry on year after year did not fail us.

- What we learnt from each patient was incorporated in improving the management plans of the centre.

- At the completion of one month of Indoor De-addiction treatment, the treated addicts were encouraged to come to the Centre daily as day patients for observations of their progress.

- Alternatively, the treated addicts were encouraged to extend their stay in the Centre. They worked as good peer educators for the new patients and this helped them to move towards a more stabilized De-addicted status.

The tremendous increase in the addicted population has compelled the state administration to increase the number of admissions in the existing de-addiction Centres.

Increase in the bed strength of the existing De-addiction- cum -Rehabilitation Centres beyond a reasonable number requires re-consideration.

- **Addicts under De-addiction treatment require intensive and broad-based care on the principle of individual-specific and situation-specific management.**

- An optimal staff/patient ratio is a must for such care. The addict goes through mood-swings, emotional upheavals periodically, and even during the same day. Enough staff strength and an optimum staff ratio should be available to manage such situations.

- **De-addiction cum Rehabilitation Centres with a limited number of beds and reasonable staff-patient ratio would be more successful. These could function locality wise for success-oriented De-addiction and meaningful sustained recovery and rehabilitation as the ultimate aim.**

Drug-abuse awareness 'Rallies' and 'Runs' and 'Pledges': These are important for general awareness and are also of motivational value for the general public to stay drug-free.

Awareness rallies and runs are essential in the present scenario of widespread drug-addiction; the practical value of many such well-intentioned efforts require dispassionate comments (from my own observations as follows):

- I share here the comments made by addicts under treatment in R.C.D.A.R.C. Amritsar who had attended these 'Rallies' and participated in the 'Runs'. Reviewed administrative management of these appears to be necessary.

- The addicts who attended these rallies confessed that they were always very keen to join such events singly or in peer- groups. Most often they found these events as good opportunities to attract some willing youth in the crowd to join their existing peer-groups of the addicts.

- The De-addiction camps held for diagnosing and de-addiction treatment, gave them similar ample opportunities to attract and convince others, to join their existing addict peer groups.

- Those in-charge of the awareness programmes are suggested to take note of my observation regarding these **to reasses their value.**

- Indoor De-addiction treatment in the Centres requires consecrated efforts. An integral approach to treatment and rehabilitation is necessary. For **amy success-oriented programme, it must be accepted that a proper understanding of the disease of addiction is**

required because the addict is helpless towards his own self.

- In brief, an addict is a victim of unfavourable circumstances, moving towards his fatal end. He cannot help himself. He remains prone to relapses. We have to intensify our efforts to help him and prevent relapses.

The occurrence of relapse/relapses is a major contributory factor towards the continued rise in the addicted population

Prevention of relapses after de-addiction treatment is mainly the responsibility of the doctors who must ensure an adequate and appropriate De-addiction treatment and sustained recovery and rehabilitation of the treated addict.

The Ministry of Social Justice and Empowerment M.S.J.E. New Delhi , recommends a minimum of one-month Indoor De-addiction treatment.

Family support is an essential factor for:-(a) Motivating the addict and keeping him agreeable to stay in the Centre for complete treatment regime. (b) Co-operating with the treating centre staff for: (1) after-care at home and follow-up visits to the Centre for one year.

In view of the mandatory recommendations of Ministry of Social Justice and Empowerment to keep the treated addict under observation for one year ;the practical value of measures such as 'DRUG VS DRUG' by the state administration (wherein the role of addicts 'Drug-Free for two months only) cannot be expected to be fruitful and successful.

Our aim in a De-addiction Cum Rehabilitation Centre should be to bring out the real personality of the addict to the forefront. These unfortunates are the victims of a highly 'drug-polluted' environment.

The Medical Faculty in general and those doctors who are treating addiction cases in their practice have a great responsibility of providing appropriate De-addiction regimes to minimize relapses and contribute positively towards a reduction in the addicted population.

The prevalent view that the lack of employment opportunities is one of the major causes is only a half-truth. Many of those employed lose their employment after starting on drug-abuse. A full chapter on this subject is included in the Book.

Acknowledgements

The complete write up in this compilation, the observation details, data analysis, the conclusions and inferences drawn from these, are all based on my experience in The Red Cross De-addiction-cum Rehabilitation Centre R.C.D.A.R.C.Amritsar . The records were maintained personally by myself as Project-in-charge and a full-time Administrator, guided by the Doctor-in-charge, and the Counsellors; in The Red Cross De-addiction cum Rehabilitation Centre. Indian Red Cross Society District Branch, Amritsar. All expressions of acknowledgement and gratitude are on behalf of (R.C.D.A.R.C.) which provided the opportunity to study the problem of DRUG-ADDICTION, THE ADDICTS, and their management. Before I was asked to take charge of the Centre as Project Director, Mr. Kapoor was the Administrator. Mr. Kapoor was a sagacious elderly person ; he was an asset to the Centre who instilled confidence in the addicts to get admitted for treatment. The Centre owes its successful start to Mr. Kapoor's approach and efforts.

The Red Cross De-addiction cum Rehabilitation Centre, Amritsar. came into existence on the initiative of Mrs. Poonam Sidhu (ITS.) Chair Person, who visualised the necessity for it at that time as well as for the future, and this was endorsed by The President, Indian Red Cross Society, Amritsar, Mr. Karanbir Singh Sidhu (IAS), the then Deputy Commissioner Amritsar. The smooth take-off of this

Centre, its sustenance and maintenance for the next two years, and its progressive leaps in the service for the addicts were all due to the goodwill and helpful concern of the Chair Person. I acknowledge with gratitude all the support and consideration given by her.

My efforts as Project Director - cum - Administrator, towards appropriate and meaningful care for De-addiction and Rehabilitation Programme gained further momentum during the tenure of Mr. K.S. Pannu as President of R.C.D.A.R.C. Amritsar. His confidence in my decisions for the management of the Centre provided the right environment for furthering integral care of the admitted addicts and the follow-up and after care. When the Centre was abruptly closed at the end of 2010 for reasons best known to the administration , the President allowed extension of Indoor treatment for completion of mandatory period for Indoor care of the admitted addicts. The President also allowed preparation of the Compilation Mannual on addiction (now a Book) from all the records personally maintained by me and the Doctor-In-charge.

Dr. J.P.S. Bhatia. a psychiatrist (M.D. In psychiatry) and Doctor in-charge of the medical care of the admitted addicts has been the main anchor for the successful services of the Centre rendered to the addicts under treatment. Enough cannot be said in recognition of his contribution to the treatment of those who became "drug-free" and are now leading a normal life. The long period of service provided by him to the victims of addiction by the Centre, from the year 1995 to 2010/11 , was possible with his unfailing regularity in attending to the indoor patients, his expert handling of all medical problems of the addict including the concurrent psychiatric disorders. He gave his services with concern and dedication. All through the entire period, his services were voluntary (except for about two years period, when the grant-in-aid was sanctioned by The Ministry of Social Justice and Empowerment (MSJE) New Delhi. **He also pioneered and practiced the concept of long term follow-up medical care along with complimentary counselling sessions for the addicts after their discharge from the Centre.This is the most beneficial and praiseworthy contribution towards addiction menace and the fact that this continues for the patients treated in R.C.D.A.R.C. while Dr. Bhatia is in his private practice. It needs to be added with emphasis that follow-up care and counselling is an absoulutely essential component for a success oriented De-addiction-cum-Rehabilitation regime.**

The counsellor Miss Prarthana (M.A. Psychology) made a notable contribution with her gentle and convincing counselling in motivating the addicts to complete the period of indoor stay and to come for follow - up visits. Miss Kulwinder Kaur (M.A. Psychology), the other counsellor who joined after Miss Prarthana left, did equally well and deserves expression of gratitude. **These two counsellors were followed by seven Experiential Counsellors, in batches of two or three, who added another dimension to the indoor and outdoor follow - up counselling, from their personal experiences of having been addicts and becoming "drug-free" while under treatment in the Centre, and subsequently kept under observation for long**

period up to one year. This made the counselling more effective. The Centre appreciates their contribution as role models, and as a gesture of gratefulness for their own recovery.

Professional nursing with a gentle and caring attitude plays a very important role in the recovery of the addicts. Smt. Dalbir Kaur contributed her best possible, by hard work over long hours of duty, learning and practicing the ethics of conduct with the addicts and their families whenever needed, along with other duties. Her efforts and work deserve appreciation as also her continuous stay in the post 'from day one of the Centre until its closure'.

Similar appreciation is for the night ward boy Late Sh. Gurcharan Singhwho showed a remarkable capacity to manage the addicts at night; most of the addicts suffered from a variable degree of sleeplessness and restlessness, and presented very challenging moments for the night staff on duty. At this point in time when this compilation is published all his colleagues and myself express gratitude and appreciation for the departed soul.

Physical Yoga plays an important role in the recovery of addicts R.C.D.A.R.C. Amritsar is grateful to Sh. Harsh Kumar, the yoga therapist for his voluntary (mostly) services for the cause.

Sh. Sat pal worked as an able and effective guard and chowkidar at the entrance gate. He prevented the entry of addicting substances and unwanted visitors very effectively. This unmatched contribution to the recovery of addicts deserves special recognition and all the praise.

It is with a heavy heart that I add a memorial appreciation for Sh. Satpal who left for his heavenly abode a few months back. His unfailing role in maintaning the Centre sanitized against entry of 'addicting substances', undesirable visitors who carried these, and the ignorant and uncouth family members who yielded to the demands of their admitted patients. Physical search by him of the addicts who came for admission /enquiry and of the accompaning family was fool proof. The credit of the success stories of De-addiction regimes in R.C.D.A.R.C. Amritsar goes to his gentle but meticulous repeated physical search in every demanding situation.

Smt. Surjit Kaur, the cook, made it possible to send home the recovered and recovering addicts, satisfied with the diet services of the Centre and with improved health at the time of discharge. Her contribution to the good reputation of the Centre is praiseworthy.

The support of the office staff has been exemplary in maintaining continuity of the Centre through difficult periods by judicious handling and extending required support in difficult situations.

I acknowledge with gratitude unstinted contribution by my steno typist Mr. Deepak Bansal for the preparation of Contemplative Compilation Manuals and the Published Book on Drug-addiction and its management.

I do not have adequate words to express appreciation and gratitude to those generous Doctors who contributed towards making the Centre well equipped for good service to the addicts under treatment. **Amongst them, a special memorial appreciation of late DR. SHIVINDER SINGH SANDHU.** (a well-known orthopaedic surgeon) who never missed contributing the monthly donations once offered at the time of the start of the Centre; this most precious goodwill gesture came to an abrupt ending with his untimely death in an accident at a young age. For me, this has always remained a personal loss because Dr. Shivinder Singh Sandhu was a favourite student during his undergraduate career and later as a generous donor towards good management of the Centre.

Lastly, acknowledgements would be incomplete without appreciation of late Dr. D.P. Sanan F.R.C.S (Edin. U.K.) my dear husband, who donated regularly during the long initial period of financial difficulties of the Centre, and cooperated unreservedly throughout my association with the Centre and I could spend very long hours daily for the care of the addicts in R.C.D.AR.C. Amritsar for fifteen years that I served the Centre.

Introduction

Drug-addiction, chemical substance abuse, and drug - abuse are different descriptive terms for the same affliction, the disease of drug addiction. Primarily, it is a disease of the mind and the body, very persistent, very pernicious, and very difficult to treat towards complete recovery of the addict, his freedom from the grip of the addictive substance; slavery that he likes for the " joy"it gives.

The "joy" giving effect of "Poppy" was known to the Sumerians of Babylonia as early as 4000 B.C. For them, poppy was "hul" (joy) and "gil" (plant). This indicates that these ancients had recognised the pleasurable psychological effects produced by the poppy plant. The Greek word for "juice" is "opium". It was as late as third century B.C. that this was mentioned as a medically useful substance in the medical literature of that time. Historically, opium continued to be used in different parts of the world for its "joy" giving action as well as for its medicinal value.

In the beginning of the nineteenth century, a highly potent substance was isolated from opium and was named Morphine after Morpheus, the Greek God of dreams. The medicinal use of opium for dysenteries was discovered in the middle of the fifteenth century and its use as 'laudanum' continued for many centuries; later its medicinal use declined. **On the other hand, ever since the isolation of morphine** from opium, it is being used as a medicine and abused for its "psychological" effects. Its pleasure / joy-giving effect is responsible for the occurrence of 'Compulsive Urge' and its repetitive use.

Opium, morphine and the opioids like heroin, brown sugar and smack, which are semi-synthetic derivatives of morphine, are highly addictive substances. When first discovered, these substances were 'abused' by few. Over the years the abuse has increased to alarming proportions due to international trafficking of these substances and easy availability to those already addicted to it and the potential victims around them.

The brief historical preface given above is of some academic interest only. **The discovery of a "joy" giving plant by the ancients has given birth to one of the most ominous eras for the psychological and physical health of the human race.It is a formidable medical challenge that the medical fraternity is facing.** Drug- addiction has already afflicted a very high percentage of the population of this country and the number is on the rise continually through peer pressure from those already addicted.

The present picture of drug abuse is that of an epidemic gone out of control because of the difficulty in implementing perfect preventive measures against the availability of addictive substances, and also inadequate prevention of relapses. While there is a daily increase in the number of new addicts, the relapse rate of those receiving de-addiction treatments is also very high; obviously, the major reason for the latter must be the inadequacy of the present treatment regimes and programmes. This realisation must be attended to in all seriousness, and at the earliest in the fight against the Drug/Substance abuse (drug-addiction) menace.

As a pharmacologist, I taught the subject to the medical undergraduates since the year 1953. *The Text Book Pharmacological Basis of Therapeutics* by Goodman and Gilman' was the main source of my own knowledge for teaching the subject to the medical students, the medical practitioners of the future. It was later in 1995 when I was asked to manage The Red Cross De-addiction Centre, Amritsar, that I realised the poverty of my own knowledge of drug-addiction/substance - abuse and the necessity of learning more about '**addiction as a disease'**, and its disastrous effects in its victim the addicts. The psychological and physical effects are described very well in the Pharmacology Text Book as also the phenomena of the (Abstinence / withdrawal Syndrome) when the drug is not available to the addict. However, the **gap between the theoretical description in the textbook and the actual face of all the changes occurring in the addicts, made me realise the absolute necessity of learning more and still more about drug-addiction from the addicts themselves.**

The master *Text Book of Pharmacology* by Goodman & Gilman has given descriptive details of drug dependence (psychological/physical); it has also given information on non-addicting substitutes for de-addiction treatment but without necessary guidelines for practical management of a drug-addict during de-addiction treatment.

As a Project Coordinator/Project in charge and finally as Project Director-cum-Administrator of The

Red Cross De-addiction-cum-Rehabilitation Centre, Amritsar, Punjab India, I had the opportunity of establishing rapport with the addicts under treatment. This gave me the opportunity to study their behavioural changes, emotional swings, their physical distress and the challenging situations created by them. I learnt how to manage such situations. Each successive day added to the knowledge and each addict became my teacher.

The objective of this Book is manifold.

(A) To share all that I Iearnt from the addicts and their families with whom I personally spent long hours of interactive dialogues, sharing with them their life stories.

(B) The application of what I learnt for improving the management details in the De-addiction Centre in my charge and promoting it to a De-addiction- cum-Rehabilitation Centre.

(C) To communicate through this Book the challenging situations faced and how these were managed.

(D) To give details of the guiding principles observed for managing The Red Cross De-addiction-cum-Rehabilitation Centre, Amritsar.

The various chapters of this book are the outcome of personally recorded observations made during repeated interactions with the addicts and their families. **Each day was a day of learning further, and this helped in handling the challenging situations created by the addicts frequently. It is to be believed that an addict under treatment can spring such surprises at any stage of his treatment.**

I will share all that I observed; I learnt and practiced in the management of the addicts admitted for treatment. The readers will accept or reject according to the depth of their concern towards the problem of drug addiction.

The obvious need of the hour is to put in the best of efforts. The readers will notice repetitions of essentials in the same chapter and also different chapters. **The ignorance about drug- addiction and the addict is so prevalent in those around him at home and elsewhere, that in actual practice, repeated emphasis and overemphasis was the only course to break the shell of persistent ignorance / incomplete knowledge leading to delayed, inadequate and incomplete treatment, poor success and high relapse rate.**

I offer an apology to the medical fraternity if they feel that I am offering unnecessary details from their point of view. However, it still remains necessary for many, in the interest of meaningful and success-oriented De-addiction management of admitted patients.

The first few chapters and the sub-chapters are focussed on explaining drug-addiction and the addict in simple words for the benefit of all those readers who may not go on to the succeeding elaborative information.

The chapter on religious and spiritual support seeks as well as suggests the possibility of substituting "God Dependence "for drug dependence.

I served the R.C.D.A.R.C. Amritsar from the year 1995 to early 2011. This provided the practical knowledge about Drug addiction and the management of the Drug-addict during indoor De-addiction treatment, as well as during his long term aftercare and his follow-up care subsequent to his discharge from the Centre. Such practical details are not given in the Pharmacology Text Books.

Unfortunately, **drug-addiction has been recognised as a disease only recently.** It is not even listed separately in the medical curriculum as such, it does not have a place in the teaching schedules as a subject and there is no mandatory allotment of the time period for didactic teaching followed by clinical training as in the case of all other diseases. Therefore, I felt the need for sharing my practical experience of managing more than two thousand seven hundred indoor patients (addicts) and nearly seven thousand outdoor patients who came for enquiry, for follow up visits, and for after-care, from the year 1995 to 2011.

It is providential that I chose to become a Pharmacologist after medical graduation, taught the subject for nearly forty years, especially the drugs acting on the central nervous system, and gained some knowledge about the problem of drug addiction from the chapters on Opium (Opiates-Morphine and its semi-synthetic Opioids- Heroin and other related substances).

Nearly eight years after my retirement from government Medical College, Amritsar, in 1987, I was asked by the then Chairperson of Indian Red Cross Society Distt. Branch Amritsar. to take up the responsibility of managing the de-Addiction Centre started by the organisation in October 1995. I now feel that this was the second providential intervention for me to learn about this awesome disease.

During a long period of fifteen years available to me, I learnt about the far-reaching effects of this terrible disease of the mind and the body of the victim of addiction, his helplessness against his psychological compulsions, his inability to struggle out of his self created situations; all these and much more made a very deep impression on me and somewhere on the way I was motivated to put in my best efforts and help them to recover from their addiction bondage. The miserable plight of the families of the addicts further strengthened my will, my desire and efforts to improve my knowledge of drug-addiction and the drug-addict and the possible difficulties in his de-addiction treatment.

As the experience with the addicts under treatment continued, the real face of drug – addiction and the miserable plight of the addict, a helpless victim of 'Compulsive Urge' for drugs, his misery and distress of his family confronted us. The enigmatic nature of the medical challenge became clearer each successive day. The longer I worked amongst them, the more I began to feel for them. The growing urge to help them turned into a passion, an obsession to understand deeply, drug- addiction as a disease, and the drug addict for his 'Compulsive Craving' for his drug and his helplessness against it. Theoretical knowledge from the books lacked the practical details. Soon thereafter it became amply clear that there was much to learn from the addicts, their families and the environmental influences.

Appointment of Dr. J.P.S. Bhatia a psychiatrist appointed as the Dr- in- charge this was another providential intervention in the interest of Drug-addicts under treatment and the challenge of the continuous increase in the number of drug-addicts/substance abusers. Dr. Bhatia and myself both of us remained voluntary workers (except for a short period of two years when the grant was sanctioned). The centre was closed in early 2011 by The Red Cross office in Amritsar.

Both Dr. Bhatia and myself personally concentrated on every patient and their drug-addiction history, their personal and family details and daily progress during treatment. These were recorded in sufficient detail. The patients themselves became not only our teachers but also evoked our sentiments for giving them the best possible care, inculcated patience in our dealings and also for providing a confidence-inspiring environment in the Centre. All these factors added to our understanding the addicts and helping them towards recovery.

The Book has taken a long time to complete as I have been aiming at sharing all that I had learnt through experience and wanted to communicate it as completely and perfectly as possible. Then I came across the following "thoughts" and ended my chase for perfection.

"A man would do nothing if he waited until he could do it so well that no one would find fault with what he has done." CARDINAL NEWMAN.

"A little knowledge that acts is worth infinitely more than much knowledge that is idle." KHALIL GIBRAN

(Author will be donating the proceeds of Royalty to the Red Cross.)

Dr. Saroje Sanan

An Appeal to the Readers

An appeal to those who feel concerned for the 'drug/substance-abusers', their families and the addiction menace which is epidemical by now. To those who have an instinctive inclination towards social service and are also fortunate to be able to instil in it a religious fervour.

This social cause requires an indepth knowledge of the drug addiction problem, acceptance of Drug/substance abuse as a curable disease and an aim towards result oriented care of the 'drug-abusers' and prevention of relapses in them. This requires enduring patience and sustained efforts with the addict himself and his family. This alone can reduce the population of addicts.

The chapters that follow in this compilation are based on my personal observations, experiences and what I learnt while managing The Red Cross De-Addiction-cum-Rehab Centre, Amritsar where addicts were admitted for indoor treatment, and also those who attended the Centre for advice, follow up and after-care. All this was done under the guidance of the Doctor-in-Charge Dr. J. P. S. Bhatia (M.D. psychiatry) and with his collaboration as an experienced Psychiatrist who treated the addicts expertly with dedication and devotion.

This Book is an offering to the Divine Power who gave me this opportunity, guided me on the way and sustained my efforts.

Accept or reject the contents as you wish, learn if you want to or reject if you so desire, add to the contents or delete what you choose to. It is all there for your discretionary choice, all depends on your inner impulsion, your attitude and the call of the conscious for 'The Unfortunates'.

P.S. It is requested that before you make your discretionary choice, it would be worthwhile to read the few chapters/sub-chapters that follow —

(1) Preview of the basics.

(2) Life of a Drug-addict and its two sub-chapters

These are few of the windows to the factual scenario of the addiction menace and may help you in your choice between reading all or some selected chapters.

Contents

Preview of The Basics in the Chapters That Follow

This Book is an attempt to share my experiences, observations, data analysis and inferences drawn and necessary suggestions based on these, and also my personal convictions supported by regular interaction and dialogues with the drug-addicts and their families, as in-charge of The Red Cross De-addiction-cum-Rehabilitation Centre, Amritsar, from the year 1995-2010/11.

Acceptance of drug addiction as a disease is necessary and also 'understanding the drug addict as an individual', his personality and behaviour changes due to drug / substance - abuse, his interaction and relationship with his own family. The expected role of the family, and other related aspects of management of an addict during de-addiction treatment and his recovery, are dealt with in the various chapters/sub-chapters.

During interaction with the families of drug-addicts, it became increasingly clear that **'THE DISEASE' Drug- addiction / substance abuse / alcohol addiction** is very poorly understood by the concerned families, and this poverty of knowledge is responsible for delayed consultation, insufficient treatment, incomplete recovery and relapses.

In my opinion tireless effort is required to convince the family members and others, by repeated emphasis on the essential aspects of the treatment management and need of their supportive role during indoor treatment and recovery. The readers will notice repetitive emphasis in this book on the key requirements for effective De-addiction treatment, successful and lasting recovery. These are repeated in the relevant contexts in more than one chapter.

Those making efforts to check addiction menace, which is spreading like wildfire, destroying youth energy and youth population, can do so effectively and successfully only if they accept **addiction as a disease** and understand the essential components of its treatment.

The most damaging prevalent ignorance is the belief that ten to fifteen days of indoor admission is sufficient for De-addict the individual. This ignorance must be counteracted by making the public aware of the difference between "Detoxification" (achieved in ten to fifteen days) and "De-addiction"; the latter requires a minimum period of one month of indoor treatment for the addict to start the journey towards successful Deaddiction through Medical Care and repeated counselling, and helpful supplementary measures. Repeated emphasis is necessary on precautions, Do's and Dont's of the "after-care" period at home and after return to his life beyond the boundaries of home.

I am aware of the fact that repetitive emphasis on the same point exposes me to criticism. I have taken the risk because I myself had to emphasize and re-emphasize TIRELESSLY with almost each and every addict and his family to achieve successful de-addiction and recovery of the addict.

Finally, the discretion is yours to go through various chapters and then decide to accept all or partially, add more to it or modify, keep the message to yourself or convey the essential knowledge to others, with as much repetition and emphasis, for a larger interest in this struggle against the "Disease Drug-Addiction" , on currently imperfect and incomplete approach leading to relapses, which add substantially to the addicted population.

My excuse for this unconventional layout is the necessity for it in the face of a nationwide problem of drug addiction menace, its devastating effects on the victim, a problem attended to inadequately and inappropriately, and lack of emphasis related to causes and prevention of frequent relapses.

Besides the thoughts shared above, some important aspects of a De-addiction regime are consolidated in the last few chapters, such as:-

a) Miscellaneous/mandatory considerations. Some readers may not have the time and patience to go through details, such unconventional supplements, concise and consolidated may be acceptable, preferring palatable small bites, to an unacceptable and time-consuming full helping.

b) Conclusive suggestions: A Supplement

c) Inclusion of Drug-Addiction/ Substance-abuse, alcohol addiction as a separate subject in the syllabus for Medical Under-graduates in the M.B.B.S. Course.

Life of A Drug- Addict is....

A life of paradoxes!!

A riddle of opposites!!

A jumble of contradictions!!

The compulsive urge for drug abuse is a highly damaging force in the life of an addict, which disintegrates his life, his personality.

An addict is an individual with tangled emotions and unpredictable behaviour. His submissive and appeasing approach for procuring "the drug" may turn into challenging defiance. He is a coward at heart with a brave front, projecting pseudo-confidence in his capacity to start a good life but he lacks the initiative.

An addict is virtually lost to himself, thence to his family. His future is buried under the debris of his disintegrated personality. His retrieval is possible only if he is given appropriate medical care by a psychiatry expert in an environment where all those around him give him unstinted care, thus increasing his self-confidence.

A deep understanding of the personality of the addict under the effect of 'addicting drugs' is required and this is possible only with persistent and patient interactive – dialogues with each addict under treatment.

An addict lives in a world of fantasy, a world inhabited by clans of drug addicts. The addicts have uncanny bondage between them and as long as it lasts it is the strongest of all human relationships. Love for the family lurks in the background and may upsurge off and on, but always under the shadow of a compulsive craving for the drug which is persistent all the time. Ultimately the addict sacrifices himself at the altar of "compulsive drug abuse". The addict needs help to regain his pre-addiction health status. **Addiction is a disease which can be treated and should be treated.**

The approach for treatment requires adequate knowledge of personality characters of the addict before he falls prey to addiction. Individually the personality characters may be related to the family background in terms of educational and financial status. Other influencing factors are family relationships, the influence of companions at school/college and the workplace. In most instances, this knowledge also provides a clue to the reasons for drug/substance abuse.

An addict needs help to restart his normal life all over again. Each addict is a unique case and warrants individual-specific dealing, keeping in mind the above described influencing factors. Many recovered addicts have shared their recovery stories. Generalised principals and recommendations are based on this shared knowledge. In good De-addiction Centres, De-addiction programmes are planned accordingly.

Briefly, not only each addict is unique, he can present individual challenges during the course of indoor treatment due to his mood swings and changes in his attitude to De-addiction treatment, response to care facilities, and counselling. The mood swings may occur on the same day or at intervals during the entire period of stay. Each such challenge is to be dealt with deftly, keeping in mind his personality changes due to addiction generally, and those relevant to the particular addict under treatment.

A repetitive emphasis on the individual-specific approach is essential because that is the foundation of sustained de-addiction after detoxification has been achieved.

The paradoxical behaviour variants in addicts are given in detail for unique management of each addict and at any challenging juncture during the treatment.

- An addict loves his own life of drug addiction and the substance-abuse pleasure that he derives from it. He may remember his normal past with remorse and may desire to recapture it during his lucid intervals but reverts swiftly to the pleasure-giving memory of drug/substance abuse.

- He is sad as a victim of drug addiction, yet repeatedly returns to this captivity with eagerness.

- His daily routine is firmly woven around 'drug-seeking' and using it while his personal and family and social life is in shreds, these remain in the background.

- He makes promises for a drug-free life vehemently and breaks these meekly and stealthily.

- He experiences ecstasy and exaltation of the rendezvous with the 'drug' and suffers from remorse of the miserable helplessness thereafter.

- He strives to overcome the sense of guilt and uneasiness by plunging into the muddy swamp of drug/substance abuse again and again.

- His efforts for positivism are suffocated by the overpowering menacing negativism that haunts him all the time.

- His investment on the transitory drug abuse joys earns him unhappiness and ruins, as interest compounded on a daily basis.

- **The life of an addict is a pendular swing between hopes and despairs of false pleasures and real misery, punctuated with broken promises, tattered determinations, haunting memories and shattered dreams.**

- He nourishes this craving to uphold his ego and self-respect on imaginative false grandeur, while he lives draped in mental poverty and perpetual want.

- His efforts towards a commanding and dominating status amongst fellow addicts ends in a humiliating defeat and slavery of circumstances.

- An imagined heightening of self-status and feeling of expanded personality, overshadowing all else around, stations him on a shaky ladder of the climb which becomes a treacherous ascent beset with repeated falls; this way he continues on his life journey condemned by his own near and dear ones.

- He expresses his apology and respect for his parents with humility and soon thereafter confronts them aggressively and violently.

- He yearns to be loved and accepted by his family. When driven by the COMPULSIVE DRUG-URGE, he rejects them and their caring gestures with abrupt and rude behaviour.

- His trading with DRUG/SUBSTANCE-ABUSE is a barter of loss between drug-dependent pleasure and relief from withdrawal misery, set against grief, anxiety and poverty.

- **In his lucid moments, the addict prays to God, for freedom from addiction and often, soon thereafter he pleads to the Almighty for a quick supply of "His-Drug".**

- He may have a short transitory period of powerless thoughts to reject 'drugs', and soon thereafter he accepts 'drug' offer willingly and with tenacity.

- **The saddest paradox of the life of an addict is that when he had the mind power to reject the offer of addicting substances, he became a victim of unfavourable circumstances, and his enslaved will became powerless. As a victim of addiction, either he has no will or has some flickering shadows of the same, bereft of its executive power. Ironically, when all those concerned about his welfare awaken to his helplessness, they still expect him to exert the will power that he does not have.**

The Journey Of The Untreated Drug-Addict Towards Normalcy Becomes One, Without A Beginning, And With A Lost End — The Only Hope Lies In Expert Medical And Psychological Care, Unstinted Support And Care By The Family And Understanding By All Those Around Him.

Finally, all those who know an addict and those who want to help him, work for him or work amongst the addicts, should be aware of the reality picture of an addict, a generally condemned person.

Fifteen years of experience as Project-in-Charge /
Project Director/Administrator in The Red Cross De-
addiction-cum-Rehabilitation   Centre   R.C.D.R.C,
Amritsar, enabled me to understand the victims of
the "Disease Drug-addiction" , through long hours
spent in interactive dialogues with them and their
families.

1.2

The Drug-Addict Speaks for Himself and He Pleads

- I am a victim of Drug-addiction/Substance-abuse, disliked, rejected and shunned by old friends and my own family.

- I am told that Drug-addiction is a disease and it is treatable. I implore for your help because I cannot help myself. Please De-addict me appropriately towards a sustained recovery so that I am able to recapture my old self. I will share some truths about myself.

- I love my family. During the short lucid intervals that I have in between two intakes of the abuse-substance. I enjoy being drug-free, I make promises with my own self to remain drug-free and uphold my head high, rejoin the mainstream of life, regain employed status, resume my business activities/studies/earlier profession.

- **Unfortunately, I remain unaware of the urge for drug-abuse persisting somewhere in the depths of my consciousness (I am told it is the sub-consciousness).**

- The experience of being drug-free during the lucid intervals is a superficial freedom. 'The urge' for taking the drug lurking in the subconscious 'upsurges' when the effect of the previous dose is over.

- **My promises are shattered and the craving for the next dose of the addictive substance reappears as an irresistible Urge.**

- **We addicts always live under the shadow of a 'Compulsive Urge' even after receiving de-addiction treatment. This is due to the persisting memory of the pleasurable experience of 'drug' use.**

- Insufficient Indoor stay for my De-addiction treatment is a major reason for relapses. Relapse occurs if the stay in the De-addiction Centre is short.

- My family does not follow the counselling instructions given at the time of my discharge from the Centre.

The triggering factors for the Compulsive Urge are :

(a) A mobile conversation with an old friend triggers the memory of drug-use pleasure.

(b) An unkind condemning remark by a family member about my addiction makes me feel desperate.

(c) Presence of money in the pocket tempts me to procure the 'drug' and use it.

(d) I am allowed to or compelled by the family to start working before my drug-free status is stabilized.

(e) Constant reminders by the family of my drug-abuse affliction becoming the cause of family misery.

The treating Centre and my family and other well-wishers can help me by protecting me from the above triggering factors.

Drug- Addiction / Substance- Abuse And Its Victim The Drug Addict

(An attempt to highlight the essential features of this disease and related key essentials to be observed for its successful treatment)

The alarming magnitude of "Drug-abuse" has become a matter of great worry for the households which are affected by it. Addiction has a devastating effect on the population, particularly of young India. **The youth of this country are turning into crumbling pillars of future India. If the situation which is worsening each passing day, is not accepted and not understood in its entirety and effective steps are not taken and particularly if the De - addiction regimes are not re–assessed and planned for sustainable recovery, this menace is heading towards unmanageable dimensions.**

My aim is to highlight the need for a more appropriate approach to the de-addiction regimes. My effort through this chapter is to focus on the existing lacunae in the essential awareness for the treatment of this disease.

As in the case of other diseases addiction also exhibits signs and symptoms which can help in its detection provided this knowledge is given during

the medical graduation course and this disease is detected and treated early.

'Addict' is the commonly used abbreviated form for a drug-addict, a person who takes by mouth, by inhalation or by injection the addictive substances, which make him physically and psychologically dependant on these. He is also labelled as a Drug user/Drug abuser; his condition is known as 'Drug-addiction'. Drug dependence, a more easily understood descriptive term, is neither fully correct nor comprehensive. Addiction is a state of tenacious drug dependence and the addict is miserable physically and psychologically, when deprived of the drug and has to take the drug compulsively.

An addict is that unfortunate person who is unwittingly sliding down to his self-propagating destruction. He is an individual with clouded thinking, fractured personality propped on dazzling imaginations, broken relationships, mood swings and unbridled temperament.

An addict is a sick person, badly bruised and traumatized emotionally, dejected with himself in his brief lucid moments. He is rejected by near and dear ones, treated as an outcast by his neighbours. Even his mental state is of extremes, of aggressive behaviour and of depression. Some may even have suicidal thoughts.

An addict with tangled emotions may exhibit variable behaviour and extreme mood swings on the same day. The variability of behaviour can range from submissive apologies to an aggressive confrontation. The former may be a genuine remorse or else it is a soft face hiding behind it crafty planning. The unbridled temperament is the cause of broken relationships at home and at the place of work, while his bond with the 'drug' and his peer group remains firm.

Such a person is standing on the brink of a precipice, swaying with the gusty winds of environmental addiction storm; a little push even with a verbal reprimand can push him over the edge. Any kind of physical torture makes him more obstinate for drugs. Imprisoning him in the house, and parading him in public a torture treatment narrated to me by some parents) is not only wrong but is a counter productive approach. The addict needs to be persuaded gently but firmly. He should be counselled with carefully worded positive dialogue.

The world of an addict remains confined to his drug - use and his drug - user companions and their common efforts for the procurement of the addictive substance.

Drug addiction- A Treatable Disease

Drug-addition has been 'ACCEPTED AS A TREATABLE DISEASE'. Therefore, it necessitates that the disease and its effects on the mind and the body of its victim are well understood by all those who are concerned (obligatory or otherwise) , and work for his welfare and treat him.

The disease of drug addiction / substance abuse :

The various chapters of this book deals with the different aspects of the basic personality of the addict, his behavioural changes due to drug abuse, his interaction with the family, the expected role of the family, and other related aspects of management of the addict during de-addiction treatment and his recovery.

In simple words, drug addiction is a disease of compelling desire (the compulsive urge) for its use. The disease is very persistent and pernicious in its grip on the individual. He does not seek medical help because he does not want to be deprived of the pleasure-giving effects of the 'drug' which is responsible for the compulsive urge in him. As the 'urge' increases, its fulfilment becomes the only purpose of his daily life to the exclusion of all else, his health, professional obligations, family ties, care of his children if married, care of his parents. His thoughts remain hazy and clouded and he has no clear perspective of his surroundings and life in general, He becomes a problematic member of the family, who can neither be accepted as such, nor rejected fully.

If the addict is to be helped, he is to be understood with empathy and not with mere sympathy and mechanically applied generalised rules.

This disease of "compulsive urge" for taking the addictive substances is characterized by "impulsive" responses of the addict to any surrounding situation, and in his family relationships. Because of the very nature of these changes, the addict is unable to help himself and those around him can also not do so without understanding and having an in-depth knowledge of the disease and its effect on the individual.

The addictive substances act on the Central Nervous System. In simple words, both psychological and physical dependence is due to this central action. Psychological dependence is due to the experience of 'pleasure' and 'joy' by the person after taking "the drug", and this drives him towards its repeated use, initially periodic when the desire is mild and, later when it becomes more intense, its use becomes very **'compulsive'** and more frequent. The intervals between repeated drug/substance abuse decrease with the passage of time. **This is due to an adaptive and reinforcement mechanism in the Central Nervous System.**

The "compulsive urge" which is responsible for repeated use of the drug by the addict is a very forceful urge and sustains his efforts to face risks and dangers to procure his 'drug'. The bond with the drug is above all other considerations, including the nearest family relationships. I narrate here a heart - touching incident witnessed by me. The addict, driven by his 'compulsive urge' for the drug, left the house stealthily to procure it while the dead body of his wife lay at home, and the family waited to perform the last rites.

When the addictive substance is not taken, the addict becomes very restless, suffers from lack of sleep, severe aches and pains in the legs and the back, watering of eyes and nose and vomiting and diarrhoea in some; these are collectively called the "Withdrawal" Symptoms (the "Abstinence Syndrome" in the accepted scientific terms).

The above description of the ' withdrawal symptoms' are of help in early detection of disease of Drug- addiction/Drug-abuse in an individual and serves as warning signals for the family to seek medical help for him.

Thus an addict is that unfortunate helpless individual, a victim of unavoidable surroundings and circumstances, who is unknowingly and unwillingly sliding down to self-destruction. He is unable to help himself. If the addict is to be helped, he must be treated with 'EMPATHY and not with just routine de-addiction Indoor treatment not even confirming to the Mandatory Recommendations /Guidelines of Ministry of Social Justice and Empowerment (M.S.J.E.) ; this particularly refers to those Centres where the indoor treatment is limited to02 ten to fifteen days of detoxification.

An addict is an individual with clouded thinking, tangled emotional behaviour, and fractured personality, propped on deceiving imaginations and fantasies. The family expects from him to use his will power to refuse drugs, which he is unable to do. He is condemned with words and harsh gestures and made to feel like a rejected member of the family. This does not help him.

Treatment of The Disease of Drug- Addiction / Substance- Abuse / Alcohol- Addiction

It is an obligatory necessity to overrule the attitude of stigmatizing an addict and rejecting him. This requires widespread awareness in the families and acceptance of this truth by them.

The high relapse rate is a very important factor for the unabated increase in the addicted population, in spite of laudable efforts by the administration towards restricting the easy availability of addictive substances. **In this Book, the focus is on the occurrence of relapse / relapses after treatment due to inappropriate De - addiction regimes for various reasons.**

The awareness that drug addiction is a disease, is a major step towards the possibility of a successful De-addiction treatment regime. As in the case of all other diseases, successful treatment is based on signs and symptoms, early detection and knowledge of its effects on the various body systems inclusive of mind and psychology.

Unfortunately, drug-addiction / substance abuse is not listed as a disease in the medical books and there is no detailed information on its treatment and no training schedule for its management,

therefore, it remains an enigmatic medical challenge.

Acquiring an in-depth knowledge is not only a pre-requisite but also an absolute necessity for correct and adequate treatment of a drug-addict. This compelling need can not be over-looked.

If the DISEASE of DRUG-ADDICTION is not treated properly and adequately the addict sacrifices his life at the altar of his 'compulsive drug-abuse'.

Medical treatment of this disease is the responsibility of the Medical Faculty. Only a psychiatry specialist should treat the addicts and he should ensure that the care of the addicts is in the hands of a devoted and committed team in the treating Centre.

Contrary to the view that the addict is himself to be blamed for his 'yes' to drugs, there are various predisposing causes and precipitating factors which drive him for his self - destruction through drug-abuse. Easy availability of 'drugs' is the most challenging serious problem being vigorously attended to by the concerned authorities.

It is under constraint I write that poverty of knowledge about drug addiction as a disease exists not only in the homes of the addicts, it is also there amongst many of those practicing De-addiction of drug addicts. I offer an apology for the above statement which is based on my personal perception and knowledge through inter-reactive dialogues with addicts and their families. I must also add here, that the regrettable lack of adequate knowledge is due to poverty of contents on De-addiction management in the Pharmacology Text Books. The medical graduate remains ill-equipped to treat a drug-addict appropriately. I had been a Professor of Pharmacology in Medical College, Amritsar, before I took over, as Project Co-ordinator in The Red Cross De-addiction cum Rehabilitation Centre R.C.D.A.R.C. (Amritsar) in October 1995 and finally as Project Director and Administrator. I realised the insufficiency of the knowledge that I imparted to the medical students for the treatment and management of an addict and his disease addiction.

The teaching contents on the 'disease drug-addiction' and practical training for its management await and its inclusion in the syllabus for medical graduation.

Awareness of all the aspects of this disease needs to become a widely spread message. Besides the home factors, there are many more beyond these boundaries, and there are many other avoidable and eliminable causes also which need to be attended to for more successful results of treatment and for reduction of relapses and magnitude of addiction menace.

I do hope that the required addiction awareness advice is given with repetitive emphasis by the doctors practicing De-addiction of the addicts. If they are not observing this, my humble plea to them is that they do so henceforth, for effective De-addiction treatment successful results and minimal relapses in the treated addicts.

After detection of drug / substance-abuse by a person, the treatment of the disease Drug-addiction consists of four important consecutive phases, Detoxification, De-addiction, Recovery and Rehabilitation.

Responsibilities of the family begin with early detection of drug addiction / substance-abuse in the household member:

Early detection and admission to a De - addiction centre for indoor treatment is the most essential first step towards Drug-addiction management for good recovery of the addict and for reducing the misery of the family. The responsibility lies with the immediate family.

Drug-abuse by a family member may remain undetected unless obvious changes are noticed in his behaviour. An obedient cooperative young growing child of good temperament, regular in his daily routine of going to school / college / workplace, sharing his free time with the family and putting forward his demand in a nice and polite manner and accepting refusal without much fuss, may show changes. The same child when hooked to drugs exhibits an obvious change in his behaviour and the above-described qualities of a good child are replaced by their opposites.

There are changes in the daily routines of the addict ; procuring the drug and taking it becomes his main aim and occupation of his life. Restrictions on his movements make him irritable, angry and even aggressive.

i.   A drug abuser avoids sitting with the family and avoids eye contact during conversation.

ii. A pleasant personality changes into an individual sullen in appearance, who starts remaining aloof from the family and does not share his thoughts and his movements with them.

iii. He is reluctant to share with the family, his outdoor activities and his non-purposive movements out of the house. He develops unpleasant and abrupt behaviour in response to a well-meaning enquiry. This is a common complaint by the family members when the addict is brought to a De-addiction centre.

iv. He shows increasing tendency to remain away from the house without sharing the purpose of going out and he responds unpleasantly on being questioned or else gives misleading information.

v. As he becomes increasingly involved with his peer group he spends the entire day out of his house leaving early morning and returning very late at night and avoiding meeting with his family members. The mother out pours her love and concern for him by feeding him with a nourishing diet however late at night he returns to his home.

vi. His attendance in the school/college/ workplace becomes irregular. A school/college going young addict avoids questions about his daily performance in the tests and misinforms about the dates for the parent and teacher meet and his misconduct in the school is not known by the parents.

vii. In the case of an employed addict, poor attendance at his place of employment results in pay cuts, suspension or even dismissal from service.

viii. If the addict is self-employed, obvious income reduction is noticed by the family and the addict tells false stories.

ix. An addict belonging to an agriculturist family or else himself an agriculturist, remains happy working in the agricultural farm because slipping away from there is easy and he can arrange peer group meetings for drug abuse in his own fields.

x. With the passage of time, the quantity of drug required to satisfy his Compulsive Urge increases as also its frequency and expenses incurred.

xi. An addict always remains short of money; his own earnings decline, his expenses on drugs increase and he starts stealing money, selling household things, jewellery, self-owned transport and he start selling or mortgaging property owned by him. He remains under debt mostly.

xii. **Money and jewellery snatching on the roadside, road rages and criminal activities are becoming more frequent with an increase in the addicted population. The families of such helpless offenders must remain aware of Drug-addiction as a possible reason.**

xiii. An addict assisting in the family business is able to steal money from the daily earnings; in such cases detection of his Drug abuse habit is easier.

Unfortunately, in most cases, the delay in detection is due to an unwisely caring and indulgent but ignorant mother, who plays a major role. Either she does not know the warning signs or else she does not share her suspicion. On the contrary, she conceals it from the rest of the family and concentrates on the health care of the addict with good nourishing food (incl. 'Desi Ghee'), serving it at any late hour of the night when he returns home after taking the drug. She fulfils all his demands including that of money. She does all that but does not share it with the family. Instead, she makes him promise that he will leave drugs; the addict usually makes a false promise or else he is unable to keep it because he is a victim of 'Compulsive Urge' for the abuse substance.

As addiction becomes deep-rooted , further changes in the drug user are not only more obvious but also more serious. He may join addict groups, who may provide him with the addicting substances free of cost initially and the family is unaware. As his drug/substance-abuse increases, the free supply is withdrawn and he is asked to purchase ' Drug' on his own. This compels him to demand money from his parents, friends and relatives. On refusal, he may become increasingly aggressive or even violent. Alternatively, he may start stealing money, jewellery and other household things. At this stage of helplessness against "compulsive urge", he does not hesitate to sell household items such as scooter, car at throwaway prices without any remorse. He pretends to go out to work and he meets the peer group in prefixed meeting places.

In his own house, he chooses some far off corners for taking his 'drug', interestingly in the bathing room. This information was given by many addicts themselves. Such activities are carried out in the

middle of the night when the family is asleep. The bathing room is a place of choice for abuse substances taken through inhalation by the smack users. These details are given here to educate and forewarn those families who do not know the present scene of drug-addiction and help them to save their children from becoming hardcore addicts.

Early and effective intervention by the family can save the addict from reaching the extreme stage. An individual who is getting drawn to drug – abuse requires an understanding of his disease, firm yet affectionate and friendly handling, almost twenty-four hours vigilance and confidence-inspiring dialogues with him which can convince him about the need for medical consultation and help.

The above described behavioural changes remain unnoticed, undetected, overlooked, unattended and uncared for long periods because of ignorance and lack of adequate knowledge about detection of addiction and its effects on body and mind and his behavioural changes.

As mentioned earlier also, the medical consultation and treatment are delayed due to misconceived love and indulgence by doting mother / grand parents / brother/sister, all hopeful of changing him, do great harm to the addict and to themselves.

Procuring 'the drug' by any means and taking it becomes the most important need and daily routine of the addict and all his thoughts and activities revolve around this only. If he is restricted he becomes very aggressive and even violent and may even physically harm the family. Often the family learns about his addiction at this stage.

2.4

The supportive role of the family is as important as an appropriate Medical Care:-

The family should not consider **drug addiction as a stigma but accept it as a treatable disease**. This sub-chapter focuses on the role of the family, friends and colleagues/employers at the place of work.

A drug addict becomes the cause of his own ruin and also that of the family. The parents remain miserable; many suffer from depression, heart disease or general ill-health. The children of a married addict grow up in an environment which hampers their physical and mental growth; some of them grow with personality disorders.

Home and family-related overindulgence and pampering of the growing children, for example : either allowing them free use of money or giving in to all their demands. Equally harmful is an attitude of neglect especially that of the father imposing unnecessary restrictions on minor demands.

Generally, the family is ignorant of the fact that addiction is a disease which is treatable. The family needs repeated counselling and should be convinced to have faith in the Doctor, the Counsellors and the Project in-charge. At the same time, the family should instil an attitude of trusting submission in their ward to the suggestions given by the Centre staff. An atmosphere of discord in the family and poor economic status negate the above helping factors. **Children with such family backgrounds seek relief and pleasures outside the home and in the company of undesirable persons who get them hooked on to drugs and their life remains under the influence of such a peer pressure.**

History of unattended obstinate nature and volatile temperament from early childhood, is a recognised cause of falling prey to the disease of drug / substance-abuse. Parents of such children should be counselled on this aspect.

The present scenario demands that all family members should become aware of the possibility of drug- abuse menace and they must be given counselling / knowledge to enable them to detect drug/substance-abuse habit of their ward at an early stage.

Early detection and timely treatment in a De-addiction Centre prevents long-continued use of the 'DRUG' and its hold on the addict becoming more tenacious, thus making De-addiction success more difficult to achieve.

During indoor treatment in a De - addiction Centre, the family must follow with faith and trust, all the precautions and suggestions given by the Doctor/Project in-charge. The indoor addict is always keen to cut short his stay and he may become aggressively insistent on this demand. If his pleading fails, he may try to persuade the family through complaints about food and living facilities in the centre. The principle of individual-specific approach for the addict, and family counselling are essential component of the management.

Subsequent to discharge from the de-addiction centre after treatment, the addict becomes the sole responsibility of the family, provided the Centre management has given them appropriate awareness of cautions and precautions to be observed by them to help the addict to remain 'drug-free' thereafter. These include:-

a) Total restriction on the movements of the addict beyond the boundaries of home.

b) There should be no condemning reference to his drug abuse period.

c) A caring and affectionate attitude and atmosphere should be provided in the home.

d) The family must remain tolerant of unpleasant behaviour of the addict off and on, remembering that he has had 'a new birth' of his pre-addiction life and deserves the same care as a new born.

e) Most importantly, the family should accompany him for a regular periodical check-up by the Doctor/management of the centre. Such check-ups are an absolutely essential part of proper after-care for sound and sustained recovery.

f) **The family must accept that the Doctor / Project in-charge / Counsellors are the best guides to decide when to allow the treated addict any freedom of movement and to go out to work. Early return to work, while he is still in an 'unemployable' phase after De-addiction is a major cause in most of the relapse cases; this occurs on account of the ignorance of the family. This factor is further clarified in the chapter titled, Unemployment as the cause of drug addiction.**

Responsibility of the De-Addiction-Cum-Rehabilitation Centre where the addict is admitted for treatment

Each drug-addict admitted for indoor treatment is a unique case and warrants an individual – specific approach, and if so needed it should also be situation -specific; behavioural and situational variations are very common in an addict and he can present varying challenges during the course of indoor treatment.

Up-surging of the memory of the pleasure experienced after taking the drug and non-unavailability of the abuse substance is a common cause of mood swings during indoor treatment. Unnecessary restrictive measures in the De -addiction Centres and unethical mishandling by the staff may act as provocations on a highly labile temperament of the addict under treatment, who is either emotionally or conversely a defeated, dejected, and depressed individual unable to help himself. Such frequent behavioural challenges require deft handling, keeping in mind both his personality changes due to addiction and those related to his basic temperament.

The relapse rate in those treated for drug-addiction can be reduced only when the drug-addicts are appropriately and adequately treated after the initial detoxification phase. This would be a major

positive step in downscaling addicted population. A result-oriented treatment is as important as any other measure to reduce the magnitude of addiction menace in the population.

Project in-charge / Project Director / Manager should have the essential knowledge about the addicts and the disease addiction. He / she must ensure that the serving team of the centre maintains ethical conduct, a positive and confidence-inspiring atmosphere for the addicts under treatment and provision of good nourishing diet and a healthy comfortable environment.

The difference between 'Detoxification treatment' and "De - addiction" must be well understood; these are two different phases of the De-addiction treatment regime. (The difference will be explained under Chapter- 6 Dispassionate analysis Pg 61)

During the detoxification period (usually of seven to fifteen days) the addicting substance is simply eliminated from the body and with the start of the De-addiction treatment, the urge for the addictive substance decreases gradually.

The concept that Detoxification over a period of fifteen days achieves De-addiction target is an over-optimistic expectation which does more harm than good.

Such treatment regimes have left a trail of unaccounted, unreported relapsed cases and the number of addicts continues to rise. The success of mere detoxification without extending the indoor stay for sustainable Deaddiction is presumptive and fallacious. The complete treatment regime is in terms of many months, preferably a year or more and even longer.

The important question is: Is it not the time now, however late it may be, to reassess the results of our efforts over the years, and accept as to how inadequately we have attended to the challenging problems of successful De - addiction treatment? Increase in the number of Deaddiction Centres where the addicts are admitted for seven to fifteen days for "Detoxification", without attending to the real issues of this disease, has not reduced the number of addicts in the population because ' Detoxification' is not De-addiction and relapse cases continue to be on the increase.

Not much can be achieved unless the whole staff of any De-addiction Centre is trained by the Doctor / Project Director / Manager in-charge for a well-planned treatment regime followed by fruitful, effective and result oriented after-care programmes.

Success requires a continuous conjoint effort by the doctor and his team at the De - addiction centres.

Full awareness of the distinction Between Detoxification and De-Addiction. Duration of indoor stay influences the success of treatment:

The minimum period of one-month indoor treatment recommended by M.S.J.E New Delhi is based on the fact that the treatment regime consists of two successive phases. The first phase of Detoxification treatment takes about ten to fifteen days and only rarely it needs to be longer.

During the above phase, the addict feels better physically and the well-meaning and motivated addicts make a determination to lead a "drug-free life". Detoxification makes the addict more positive during the counselling sessions, and he seeks help willingly and responds to advice. Towards the end of Detoxification phase, he becomes less demanding, his participation in 'occupational therapy' and games improves, and the Compulsive Urge subsides gradually. He becomes helpful to his fellow addicts. The second phase of the De-addiction treatment regime helps him to move towards recovery. As the duration of stay increases, self-motivation to stay drug-free also increases gradually. This facilitates his rehabilitation after discharge and good after-care at home.

The management team of any De-Addiction-cum Rehab. Centre must be fully aware of the above described difference between Detoxification and De-addiction.

To presume at the end of ten to fifteen days detoxification period that De-addiction of the addict is achieved is a serious lapse in the De-addiction programmes and plans. Unfortunately, such claims are very often made by even the most well-meaning, and practiced by genuine well-wishers.

The second phase of the De-addiction treatment regime is that of helping the addict towards "DE-ADDICTION" possible only after satisfactory detoxification has been achieved. **Counselling is the starting point from which the 'detoxified addict' moves towards recovery.**

An important point to note is that an addict becomes responsive to counselling only after he is 'detoxified' and, the 'drug' induced mental haze produced by drug - abuse and the irresistible 'compulsive urge' for use of 'drugs' is on the decline, and self-motivation to stay 'drug-free' appears and increases gradually.

CONCLUSIVELY: We have to remember that an addict in the family becomes the cause not only of his own ruin but also of his family. The parents remain miserable, may suffer from depression, heart trouble and general ill-health. This upsets the life of other members of the family. In the case of an addict who is married and has children, their misery is imaginable.

An addict requires help by many sections of the general population and the medical faculty. Success can be achieved and made more certain by:

a.) The Doctors who put in their best with whole hearted and expert professional commitment.

b.) The social workers contribute with devotion and dedication and unflinching efforts.

c.) **The public must be made aware that they should have an unbiased acceptance of drug – addiction as a treatable disease and not believe it as a stigma.**

d) The NGOs to be made aware of the responibility of giving well planned and unstinted help.

e) The government authorities can play a major role in minimizing the addiction menace by their continued and effective steps for preventing easy availability of addictive substances.

We all must move on, to achieve the best we can in our fields of activity, that we choose voluntarily or else if we are chosen for it.

Specific recommendations for the parents and other members of the family during the recovery period of the addict at home

Subsequent to a well-planned regime during, the mandatory Indoor treatment period as recommended by M.S.J.E. the support of the family during the recovery period at home plays a crucial role after the addict is discharged from the De-addiction Centre.

- An appropriate environment at home helps the addict towards an early and successful recovery.

- **The most important responsibility of the whole household is to provide a congenial home atmosphere for his recovery.**

- **Parents and other members should develop a friendly relationship with him and encourage him to share his thoughts and difficulties with them ; sharing with outsiders, particularly his old companions exposes him to risky situations.**

- **He should not be nagged and scolded for his old mistakes with a harsh and high handed approach and he should not be reminded of his role in the ruin of the family.**

- **During this period he should be given a good nourishing diet and he should be encouraged for physical activity and exercise. He should be** kept occupied with some responsible job at home and made to feel a useful member of the household. He should be motivated and helped to plan for a good future.

- Throughout the recovery period at home, the family should respect his "Drug-free status" in the household, encourage and appreciate him for his participation in family matters. These gestures help him in building up his self-confidence.

- The addict should be kept within the boundaries of home at least for the first three, preferably six months after discharge from the Centre.

- During the period at home Cell Phone should not be available to him. The cell phone is the easiest means for making unwanted contacts and availability of drugs (even one exposure to drugs / abuse substances can re-awaken the craving for it). He should not be allowed to use any transport, his own or that of the family and should not be allowed to go out.

- He should not be trusted with money and not sent out for minor household purchases; a common mistake that is made even by the most sensible families.

- After a reasonable period, he should be allowed to go out accompanied by a family member and later after suitable interval freedom of movement on his own can be allowed and periodically checked.

- Recently treated Drug-free addicts are likely to misuse this freedom. All those who returned to R.C.D.A.R.C. with a relapse confessed misusing availability of money.

- It is a folly to expect from an addict who is not appropriately De-addicted to say no to drugs by using his will power. **Unfortunately, an addict has neither the will nor the power; the will and the power to refuse addictive substances is the earliest causality of drug-abuse.**

- **Counselling of the wife of a recovering requires special mention. She should have a correct, friendly, persuasive and firm approach in keeping him away from the drugs.**

- As observed in R.C.D.A.R.C. the married addicts recovered faster. An Indian wife bestows undivided and devoted attention. **Her inexhaustible patience in spite of her husband's mistakes is helpful in successfully steering him to recovery.**

- **An addict recovering at home after De-addiction treatment should be brought to the Centre for follow-up care for six months at least, if this is done for a longer period it is more helpful. This was observed in RCDARC Amritsar.**

3

Alcohol Addiction

Alcohol is a socially accepted drink. Over the years its use has increased in alarming proportions, involving all age groups, irrespective of financial status, education level and even in defiance of religious teachings and specific restrictions by the family. In India, it has become a symbol of social status to serve alcohol in all kinds of social events and all kinds of family celebrations and other socially compulsive obligations.

Alcohol has always had a unique distinction of being a socially acceptable substance for self-induced intoxication. In the earlier days, this was a privileged sanction for the rich, and its advantage was taken by a small number. Over the years its use has increased tremendously.

In the western countries more than fifty percent adults use alcohol daily and more than ten percent of these are considered "heavy drinkers" and labelled as 'alcohol addicts'. In the present scenario of substance-abuse in India, alcohol is the most commonly used socially acceptable abused drink.

Thus, alcohol addiction occurs due to misuse / excessive use of a licensed substance. One who drinks daily, excessively and undeterred, is an alcoholic; he is an alcohol addict with a 'compulsive urge' to drink alcohol which is very easily available. An alcohol addict can purchase it in the open market, he can maintain his own stocks, he can drink it openly and defiantly in his own house, even to the point of becoming an obvious nuisance day after day. The family is unable to dissuade him while he continues to move on the path of self-destruction and also that of the family.

Alcoholism is a disease which affects all the major body systems; apart from the obvious behavioural nuisance that an alcoholic creates at home and in public places. An Alcoholic suffers from loss of appetite, digestive stomach problems, deteriorating liver function and, muscle and nerve degeneration and above all this, clouding of thought processes, and irrational behaviour.

Alcohol consumption is responsible for domestic crimes, road accidents, and public brawls. Unfortunately, the increasing tendency for alcohol drinking amongst the teenagers is posing new domestic and public/society-related problems and new areas of criminal activities. Loss of productivity in the workplaces of the addict. It is a saga of wasted lives, domestic violence and broken homes, juvenile delinquents and an increase in poverty figures.

Alcohol-abusers outnumber the abusers of other substances. All alcohol-abusers are potential drug-addicts; either they continue with alcohol only, or else they switch over to other addicted substances: quite a few become multi (poly) drug-users (inclusive of alcohol).

The problem of alcohol addiction is being addressed in the context of taking alcohol daily which may lead the user to become a ' compulsive alcoholic' progressing to alcoholism with its inevitable health hazards.

Amongst all the substance abuse problems, treatment of alcohol addiction is the most elusive medical challenge.Alcohol drinking is an easily noticeable habit and is detected early by the family, friends, work partners and employers. However, in most cases, it remains untreated. During his lucid intervals, an alcoholic is remorseful and even apologetic and repeatedly promises to give up drinking, but he is unable to overcome "the compulsive urge" and with the passage of time abuse increases in quantity and frequency of its intake.

TREATMENT OF AN ALCOHOLIC

Observations of significance with regard to the 'treatment of alcohol addicts' made in The Red Cross De-addiction-cum-Rehab Centre, Amritsar are shared here.

With a few exceptions, alcohol drinker refuses to seek advice on his substance-abuse problem. He denies emphatically that his alcohol intake is more than it should be, justifies its use as occasional and as a social compulsion. In many instances, this tussle between him and the family continues over long periods and the alcohol user does not agree for any kind of medical consultation and treatment in a De-addiction centre. The family is unable to convince him even for a visit to such a Centre.

Factually a very small percentage of alcohol-abusers come to a de-addiction centre for consultation or treatment. A still smaller percentage of those who agree to be admitted for indoor treatment ; even amongst these very few are willing to complete one month of mandatory indoor stay.

In recent years, a larger number of alcohol abusers were brought to R.C.D.A.R.C. Amritsar by the families motivated by public awareness rallies. Those few addicts who were self- motivated got admitted willingly and remained cooperative throughout the indoor stay. Such motivated and willing users are very few. Most do not get admitted, or else promise to come at a later date but do not return.

Analysis of the yearly data records maintained in the R.C.D.A.R.C. Amritsar has revealed that the admission percentage of the alcohol abusers for any admission year is the lowest amongst the total drug-abusers admitted for indoor treatment.

In a large number of cases of drug addiction, alcohol is the 'initiating abuse substance' before the person gets addicted to other drugs. However, in the multi (poly) users the incidence of alcohol addicts is less than that of the capsule and smack/heroine abusers but much higher than that of the other components such as Afeem, Injections, Syrups, Bhang, Lomotil and Alprax.

There is yet another complicating aspect in the treatment of alcohol-abusers; the treated addict (multi or single 'drug-user) starts on alcohol during the after-care/recovery period at home, by his own choice. It is also allowed by the family and even suggested by them. This is due to lack of proper knowledge. **The family must be made fully aware with emphasis, against this mistaken belief that allowing alcohol consumption will keep the addict away from the other drugs. It should be emphatically made clear to the family during counselling, and at the time of discharge that continuing with alcohol will lead to a relapse of drug abuse sooner or later.**

Alcohol as a component of multiple substance abuse poses a problem in the Recovery and Rehabilitation of multiple drug users.

There are many reasons for this. Alcohol is easily available, and for treated addicts it becomes an acceptable substitute both to the addict himself and also to his family, who in their total ignorance of the harmful potential of this substance, not only allow its use but in many cases, even themselves encourage it as a good substitute for the other addicting substances.

The problem of 'alcohol abuse' requires focus on several aspects related to this malady and its several fallouts. Most importantly, the fact that this socially acceptable drink is considered a harmless habit and is a necessity for social participation, may ultimately end up as a 'Compulsive Urge' for daily use; leading to increase in frequency and quantity of alcohol and ultimately make the person an 'alcoholic'.

Equally important is the fact that alcohol abuser who has been treated for addiction; even if he continues taking alcohol as an occasional drink, more often than not, it leads him back to the

addicted state - a relapse of the disease alcohol-addiction.

The most disturbing facts related to alcohol abuse are:

(a) its use by school and college going children.

(b) its free use in social functions where the young of the gathering are also allowed this privilege.

(c) uninhibited drinking of alcohol by the high society ladies is also on the increase and its individual, family related and social fallouts are obvious.

The daily wage earners, the farm workers take alcohol to increase their work efficiency, while some of them take it after a tire some day and some to drown their sorrows and anxieties. **Whatever may be the reason for starting on alcohol, its potential of going on to a state of alcoholism cannot be ignored. This is not an over statement for the obvious reason that alcohol is a stress-relieving and pleasure producing substance. It is easily available and is a socially acceptable home remedy, for stressful situations and for which no medical prescription is required.**

It is emphasised again, even at the cost of repetition that every alcohol user is potentially vulnerable to go on to a state of its "compulsive use/abuse on account of the above-described reasons. This should leave no room for doubt that it is an obligatory yet an enigmatic treatment challenge and requires a focussed re-assessment of what is being done and achieved, and a lot more that needs awareness and planning on family counselling, on potential hazards of alcohol-abuse especially by the very young population and growing children.

On account of my deep concern for theaddicted population, I mention my views on a glaring impropriety that I witnessed in some of the "*nukkad naataks*" staged in the awareness programmes for the public. Unfortunately, in these programmes 'Addiction' was depicted by choosing alcohol as the abuse substance, the abuser was shown as an unruly, rowdy and comical person with a staggering walk, irrational talk,irresponsible gestures and behaviour. **In short as a jocular figure, the crowd responded with laughter and fun, enjoying it as a 'Tamasha'. The intended message for the public was lost for most of the audience, except for few viewers, and only a small number 'may' have gone home with the impact of the serious aspect of alcohol addiction menace which is ruining an increasing number of households each successive year.** The real aim of such a programme is overshadowed; the real message is not conveyed and its importance is lost.

Incidence of alcohol addiction in the addicts admitted for indoor treatment from the year 2002 to 2010

1.) Only Alcohol users

2.) Multi (Poly) users inclusive of alcohol

Year	2002	2003	2004	2005	2006	2007	2008	2009	2010
1.)	4.34	33.3	3.33	11.11	12.50	4.25	1.31	8.86	8.50
2.)	51.23	43.3	41.77	50.50	55.23	37.10	58.91	58.20	57.50

Each year the admission percentage of only alcohol addicts is much lower than of those in the Multi (Poly) users. The low percentage of only alcohol users indicates the unwillingness of the alcohol addicts to be admitted.

Treatment of the disease of alcohol-abuse (addiction) is similar to that of any other substance-abuse, requires family support in detection, early medical consultation, treatment and after-care. Only a psychiatry specialist can best handle cases of both habitual alcohol users and alcohol addicts.

The public is generally ignorant of the health hazards of drinking alcohol and is unaware of its addicting potential.

An alcohol user can not be easily dissuaded to give up drinking; he cannot be convinced and is also not ready to give up his social obligations which are used as a pretext to remain in the company of likeminded therefore continues with his drinking routine. **Awareness programmes need to be planned with families in small groups in various localities, in schools and colleges with the participation of the teachers and parents.**

If the youth of the country has to be saved, priority to such awareness programmes is a must for the teaching institutions, not just occasionally but scheduled for regular and repeated exposure to counselling on this subject to awaken in them their self-determining will power.

The target for a successful De-addiction is a sustained recovery and rehabilitation without relapses. This is far more difficult to achieve in alcohol addicts compared to other substance abusers. The various reasons are given with sufficient clarity and emphasis earlier in the preceding paragraphs. Ultimately, the family can help an alcohol addict with the expert advice of **psychiatry/ addiction** expert to overcome the necessity of drinking. The responsibility of the treating centre is to explain to the family with emphasis and clarity during Indoor treatment and at the time of discharge of the treated addict.

Medical treatment of alcohol addiction:

Disulphiram (Antabuse) is the specific medicine for the treatment of alcohol abuse. It accelerates the breakdown of alcohol in the body to a substance producing a very unpleasant reaction in the person which discourages him to take the drink; the reaction includes lowering of blood pressure which may be severe enough to endanger life, and death can occur due to cardiovascular collapse.

This medicine was introduced in 1940, it is still in use. Because of the possibility of its severe toxic side effect search continues for safer substitutes. It is not curative, the treatment should be given in a hospital by a doctor aware of its life-endangering toxicity. It is hazardous to prescribe this medicine, even in small doses as maintenance treatment for use at home. The risk of serious reactions cannot be overlooked and all necessary precautions must be observed and this must be followed by a prolonged after-planning.

In Conclusion: Potential hazards of alcoholic drinks must never be overlooked by the **user, his family and his well-wishers.** Awareness programmes, timely intervention, advice and counselling, family understanding and support, education of the user about the health hazards, effects on family life, his work capacity, efficiency and also its damaging effect on his reputation. Awareness counselling of all these is expected to support his self-motivation, and a prolonged after-care 'may' ultimately reduce the 'compulsive urge' for the alcoholic drinks.

4

Counselling of An Addict
- -

Counselling is an integral part (necessary to make a whole complete) of helping an individual who is a victim of ADDICTION. Such an individual needs help at many stages and in many situations:

(1) When the family suspects or detects and he is to be motivated to take medical advice/treatment.

(2) During indoor treatment after he is admitted in a De-addiction/De-addiction-cum-Rehabilitation Centre.

(3) At the time of discharge from the Centre.

(4) During the 'after-care 'period at home or in the Centre (if the stay is extended beyond one month)."

(5) At the time of follow-up visits of the treated addict to the Centre he should be accompanied by his family for such visits.

Counselling at these different and successive stages is the joint and collaborative responsibility of the family and in the Treatment Centre (of the Dr. in-charge, the qualified Counsellors and the Project-in-charge as Co-ordinator/Director /Administrator).

Before proceeding with comments on the requirements of meaningful counselling at various stages which was practiced in (R.C.D.A.R.C), Amritsar.

Dictionary meaning of the term 'counselling' is given below:

The word counselling means — (1) Advice or recommendation. (2) Give professional help and advice to someone with a psychiatric or personal problem. (3) Process in which professional help is given for emotional or psychological problems.

The word 'professional' also requires clarification in the context of counselling of a DRUG- ADDICT under indoor treatment. **Professional (ref. 2 above) means — competent, experienced, trained, efficient, able, conscientious, knowledgeable, proper, proficient and adept.** The alternative meaning of the word 'professional used as an adverb' was applicable to some of the staff members of R.C.D.A.R.C. Amritsar and has been given to highlight the role of the other staff of the centre besides the Doctor, Project-in-charge and qualified Counsellors. **The word professional became applicable to those who participated in the care and management of indoor patients as part of their duties and imparted situation-oriented counselling.** This was possible in R.C.D.A.R.C Amritsar as each worker was trained and guided for the same.

Meaningful counselling is that which convinces and motivates the addict and makes him agreeable to deviate from perceptions and reactions of his addicted state, and helps him towards normalcy. This is possible if the **Counsellor interacts with the**

addict and understands him as an individual and his personality prior to his drug-abuse.It may appear as an easily achievable simple goal. In actual practice, it is not so. An addict becomes self-centred, evasive and a cunning and manipulative individual who evades eye contact during dialogue. To know his personality needs repeated attempts for a meaningful dialogue with him, to understand him as an individual against his family background. For a qualified counsellor this approach is not difficult to understand and apply, and experience with each addict becomes an improving step.

A commitment towards the cause of each addict, patience stretched to the maximum and Empathy, all these are essential helps. This forms the basis for individual-specific and situation-specific approach in counselling sessions with the individual alone or with the family. In this context it is necessary that the same counsellor deals with the addict throughout his stay in the Centre.

It is pertinent to add in this context the advantages of employing, "drug-free" addicts treated and kept long enough under observation in the Centre; these are approved as experiential counsellors by the Ministry of Social Justice and Employment M.S.J.E., New Delhi. Most often these counsellors have a more convincing individual-specific and situation-specific and an empathic approach which is necessary for effective communication with the addicts under treatment.

Counselling is a continuous effort over a long period during all the phases of treatment to ensure sustained successful Recovery and Rehabilitation.

Ideally, it should continue for very long after the addict under treatment is believed to have been De-addicted. Continuous family support with patience contributes towards sustained recovery and enhanced possibilities of prevention of relapses, benefiting both the individual addict and his family.

5

The Recovery Period (Vulnerability To Relapses, Cautions And Restrictions To Be Observed To Prevent These)

The disease of drug-addiction / substance-abuse is such that the treated addict remains vulnerable to relapses if the suggested precautions are not observed by the family after he is discharged from the centre and the recovering addict is not managed appropriately while at home.

During the recovery period at home, the treated addict should remain within the boundaries of the home for the first six months at least and during this period there should also be an absolute restriction on the use of his personal cell phone. It is advisable that his cell phone should not remain with him. The cell phone is the easiest way for unwanted contacts for arranging the availability of drugs. The recovering addict at home must remain protected against the availability of addiction promoting substances. Even one exposure to these drugs / substances during the vulnerable recovery period can induce a craving for further usage. It becomes more difficult to control him after re-exposure to drugs and occurrence of relapses and return of the "Compulsive Urge".

The most important responsibility of the whole household is to provide a congenial home atmosphere for his recovery when the addict returns home after treatment. He should be given all love and care that he has so far remained deprived of, on account of his addiction.

(a) He should not be nagged or scolded for his mistakes, his role in the ruin of the family, the sufferings of his parents/wife/children and all the problems faced by his near and dear ones.

(b) The family should encourage him and help him to plan a good future.

(c) The parents should keep a friendly relation with him so that he can share his thoughts, feelings and difficulties. This helps him to unburden his problems with the right persons and not seek help and advice from friends and elsewhere which always exposes him to risky situations.

(d) During his stay at home, it is for those close to him to make sure, that he is kept occupied with some sort of responsibility at home and made to feel a useful member of the family.

(e) In case he is married, has children, he remains happily occupied with them.

(f) During this period of stay at home, he should be given a good nourishing diet and must be encouraged for physical activity and exercise.

An important caution : - The recovering addict should not be trusted with money. Sending him out for household purchases to a nearby shop in the neighbourhood is a very common mistake by even the most well-meaning and sensible families, who otherwise follow all the other precautions.

Above caution is re-emphasized against this relaxation, there is a possibility that the addict will misuse this freedom. All the treated addicts who returned with relapse, have confessed misusing this freedom given to them.

The recovering addict is not to be blamed because during this period the 'De-addiction status' is still in the phase of improving gradually. Sustained De-addiction, which means freedom from "Compulsive Urge", takes months and even years to be achieved.

The fact of his vulnerability to relapses is not commonly believed and accepted easily by the family because they have not been informed about it with sufficient emphasis. As a result, the recovering addict is criticised and blamed if he relapses; for which he is not responsible.

He himself may not be happy with his downslides which occur in spite of his good intentions. The family should encourage him by believing him and, giving him verbal support in order to increase his self-confidence while still remaining vigilant. Affectionate handling by a parent or a friendly brother/sister or a sensible wife helps him towards a successful recovery and stay drug-free.

A simple but very effective suggestion for the family to help their ward to overcome his impulsive or "compulsive desire" is_: he should be encouraged to share its occurrence unhesitatingly, and the family can help by accepting it calmly and by diverting his attention towards some other issue or some such work that can interest him and also keep him occupied.

A unique method is suggested to help the addict to strengthen his own will power. He should be motivated to do some such work at home which he does not like to perform or may even dislike. Practicing this even if once daily helps him towards building up his denial to 'drug urge'. It has the desired result. **This is a psychological exercise which if done repeatedly, builds up mental will power in the same way as physical exercise builds the muscle power in spite of initial denial by the physical capacity of the individual.**

In those cases in which the family has observed the above precautions and followed all the suggestions without failing, the recovery progresses satisfactorily even in the first month at home ; he can then be allowed to go out accompanied by a mature member of the household. This further helps to build the self-confidence of the addict and keeps him happier and makes him more cooperative to stay at home for the required remaining recovery period.

The initial period of above restrictions is followed by giving him small responsibilities such as allowing him to keep small amounts of money with him and also allowing him to use of cell phone to contact his relatives and his friends, all this should be done under unabated vigilance and supervision. After a suitable interval, and as his behaviour and relationship with the family improves and when there are no obvious signs of craving for the drugs, he may be allowed more freedom to go out for a restricted time period after knowing from him the purpose of his going out and the destinations. These should be checked in a pleasant and acceptable manner.

All through his recovery period at home all the members of the household should respect his status in the family and appreciate his participation in family matters. All these gestures help him in building his self-confidence and his recovery.

In the case of a recovering addict who is married, the wife has to understand the importance of the above-given suggestions. The wife has to exercise far greater patience than any other family member. In Red Cross De-addiction-cum Rehab Centre, Amritsar, the married addicts were observed to recovered better, provided the wife followed the suggestions and precautions patiently and as long as required. **Undivided and devoted attention that an Indian wife bestows in our Indian households and her almost inexhaustible patience in spite of her husband's mistakes have been observed to successfully steer him to recovery. This highlights the importance of a persevering and patient handling of a recovering addict.**

On the other hand young unmarried recovering addicts are advised against marriage for a minimum period of one year. Very often it is difficult to make the family agree on this point.

While the treated addict is recovering at home he should be regularly brought for a check-up at the Centre from where he has been discharged ; initially once a week preferably up to atleast three months. If such visits continue much longer it is more helpful.

The addicts treated by Dr. J.P.S. Bhatia, Doctor in-charge of The Red Cross De - addiction cum Rehab Centre Amritsar, had a distinct advantage of attending follow-up meetings held weekly in his clinic. **The weekly exposure of an addict to this follow – up treatment during his recovery, proved to be of great value in ensuring sustained De-addiction.** Thus many addicts treated in the Red Cross De-addiction Centre, Amritsar have had a distinct advantage of this additional Medical care and exposure to Counselling during the recovery period; in such cases long term freedom from drug abuse up to five years and even more, as assessed through follow-up telephonic calls, can be attributed to this additional Medical Care. This assessment is based on confirmation by the family of the addicts in all such cases.

There are many factors which determine successful indoor de-addiction treatment. The primary and the most important factor is sufficiently long indoor stay subsequent to initial successful 'detoxification' which generally takes about ten to fifteen days.

Ministry of Social Justice and Empowerment (M.S.J.E. New Delhi / Chandigarh) recommends a minimum period of one month stay for indoor treatment after discharge from the Centre. The initial phase of successful De-addiction of the discharged addicts can be judged by telephonic follow up at intervals and enquiry of his drug-free status from the family. **Information given by the addict himself is not relied upon.** Telephone calls are repeated once a week and family advised to bring their ward to the Centre for regular follow-up visits.

The most important influencing factor for good recovery is the duration of indoor / in-house treatment, as determined by the length of the drug-free period after discharge from R.C.D.A.R.C Amritsar .

In the data analysis table below expressed as a percentage of the total admissions of the year:-

Duration of indoor stay is categorised in four groups. (1.) Drug-free (DF) status is analysed on the basis of minimum period of six months.

Observations in R.C.D.A.R.C. Amritsar from the year 2003 to 2010. Duration of stay grouped as follows:-

A.)   Up to 10days.   B.)   11 to 15 days.

C.)   16 to 20 days.   D.)   21 to 30 days

Abbreviations in the table: DIS (duration of indoor stay in days), DF (% of those who became "Drug – free"). **** FMTC (Follow-up Medical Treatment and complimentary Counselling) pioneered by Doctor Bhatia In-charge R.C.D.A.R.C. Amritsar in his clinic.

Year	(1 To 10 days) DF%	(11 To 15 days) DF%	(16 To 20 Days) DF%	(21 To 30 Days) DF%
2003	23.7	68.8	70.6	100% *****
2004	26.3	38.3	53.5	70.70%
2005	32.2	37.5	54.1	68.12%
2006	38.8	56.5	56.5	72.82%
2007	50.0*	55.5	68.7	80.34%
2008	29.0	44.4	75.0	80.88%
2009	33.3	57.1	70.0	79.23%
2010	24.0	54.0	62.5	82.8%
RANGE	23.7-50.0	37.5-68.8	53.5-70.6	68.12-100

***** A vigilant family observed all additional precautions advised by the Centre and 90% addicts in this group received FMTC.

1. A long duration of stay in the treatment centre gave the best recovery results.

2. Supplementary supportive effect of (FMTC), a follow-up care .

- In the year 2003 even though only 5% had stayed for 10 days. 23.3% remained drug - free, possibly due to the fact that 90% of the addicts had received FMTC. The relapse rate in this group was 8 to 14%.

- In group B 69.4% received FMTC and the drug-free were 68.8% and relapse occurred in 7.8%. Both duration of stay and FMTC were supportive .

- In group C 37.5% received FMTC and 70.6% were drug-free and relapse occurred in only 8.82%. Longer duration of stay was supportive.

- In group D with an indoor stay period of 21 -30 days even though only 33.3% had received (FMTC 100% remained drug-free, possibly both the long indoor stay and FMTC played a complementary role).

6

A Dispassionate Analysis of the Ascribed and Generally Accepted Causes of Addiction as Announced and Pronounced from Platforms of Awareness Programmes on Addiction Menace

----

Rampant availability of addictive substances is the most obvious and universally accepted cause, **laudable administrative efforts** are directed towards preventing it with multi-faceted plans: a very difficult goal to achieve in spite of laborious and multi-pronged measures, particularly in Punjab with porous borders around it.

The second most considered cause is unemployment, particularly amongst the younger generation which is presently the most vulnerable age group falling prey to Drug-abuse.

There is an equally important third factor or cause, not received due importance and attention. It is inadequate, inappropriate and unsuccessful De-addiction regimes of the treated addicts , therefore the De-addicted individuals remain highly vulnerable to relapses. Such relapsed cases not only sustain the existing immensity of the addicted population but also contribute to the aggravation of the menace: (1.) As a nucleus for peers around them (2.) By eroding the faith of the family of the treated addict and general population at large, in the success of De-addiction regime and the treating Centres.

In the light of the third factor, a dispassionate assessment should be done of the functioning of the De-addiction Centres and the De-addiction regimes followed there. In the ultimate analysis of the prevailing causes, many De-addiction Centres are needed to deal with the swelling addicted population; therefore an intense focusing on appropriate De-addiction treatment regimes is the need of the times.

The major responsibility of an ideal De-addiction treatment lies with the Medical Faculty, (the doctors' in-charge of the centres) and also a supportive family of the addict.

While awareness rallies and announcements by the concerned authorities have their own importance and value; De-addiction - recovery and rehabilitation of the addicted population requires success oriented treatment regimes in the Centres. The much emphazised role of unemployment as suggested is discussed in sufficient details in the chapter that follows.

7

Unemployment As The Basic Cause Of Drug / Substance Abuse - Employment A Panacea
----

(RELATIVE RELEVANCE OF THE ABOVE ANALYSED)

It is widely believed that unemployment is a very important contributing factor in the drug/substance abuse by an individual. Increase in employment opportunities is believed to be the panacea for this malady which is devouring the young population and is responsible for the tremendous increase in the number of drug addicts. Such views are put forward by all those who realise the gravity of the problem of substance abuse and plan for tackling the drug-addiction menace by increasing the job opportunities.

This perception that unemployment is a major cause of drug addiction and that providing employment opportunities is a much needed preventive measure to check the increase in the number of drug addicts, requires a proper analysis of the relevance of lack of occupation and unemployment, to the fast increasing 'drug-addiction ' menace and its treatment management.

Analysis has been done from the histories of the drug-addicts recorded at the time of enquiry for medical help, and at the time of admission of 'the addict' in The Red Cross De-Addiction cum-Rehabilitation Centre (R.C.D.A.R.C), Amritsar Punjab. Information was recorded as given both by the addict himself and confirmed by his family separately; as answers to the leading questions regarding the employment status, particularly in relation to the duration of addiction before coming to the De-addiction Centre.

Before proceeding with the analysis of the recorded data, it is pertinent to understand the Oxford Dictionary meaning of the words 'employment' and 'unemployment' and as it is applicable to a 'drug addict' while he is continuing with drug-abuse and during the 'after – care' period at home subsequent to his de-addiction treatment and discharged from the Centre. **Relative relevance of employment in the prevention of drug addiction and its role in the recovery of the addict, and unemployment as the cause of addiction needs to be re-assessed.**

Employment (One's Regular Trade or Profession)

Un–Employment (Lacking Employment Out Of Work, Out Of Wages)

In the context of a 'drug addict', his recovery and his recovery period, the exact meaning of the above two and other related terms also need to be known in order to understand correctly, the relevance of employment and unemployment in 'drug-addiction' and its treatment.

Employ :- Keep Busy/Occupied, One-Self Or Others.

In the case of a 'drug addict' during his after-care and his recovery period at home the responsibility lies with the family or the employer, and of the Centre in those few cases who have an extended indoor stay.

An unemployable person is unfit by character,by age or 'otherwise'

(a) treated /de-addicted addict remains 'unemployable' for a long duration, a very important consideration for prevention of relapses). Untimely, employment exposes the treated addict to risk of recurrence/relapse.

The ominous increase in 'drug-addicted' population, especially the youth, is ascribed to the unemployed young. Therefore, the repeated emphasis during awareness programs, on the need for increasing employment opportunities for them. **This concept has its own utility and it benefits some addicts, that too only when applied for the treated addicts with proper understanding and is timed properly on an individualspecific basis.**

Drug-addiction / substance abuse itself is an important factor for the rise in the number ofunemployed because drug addiction itself makes the employed individuals "unemployable" with the passage of time. The work efficiency of the individual decreases as a result of Drug-addiction / substance abuse. Those in government or private service before starting on 'drugs' get suspended or they are dismissed from service if they start on addicting substances.

Those working in the family business or on the family farm, work inefficiently after starting on 'drugs' or lose interest in the work altogether , remain absent from the workplace or even misuse the same for taking drugs/substance abuse away from the sight of the family. Majority of drug-addicts in rural Punjab, belonging to agriculturist families cannot be categorised as unemployed. Their self-occupation facilitates drug / substance abuse by them.

If a self-employed individual starts on drugs, he continues to do so for long periods because he remains self-supporting for his drug-expenses as well as for his family demands, till such time that he becomes badly incapacitated on account of his addiction or if it is detected because of his behavioural changes. **Co-existence of self-employment and addiction is supportive of the continuation of addicted state.**

In the light of what has been said above, an exaggerated emphasis on unemployment as the reason for the spread of Drug-addiction / substance abuse menace becomes a misleading concept. **As explained earlier, at any point of time, a large number of unemployed drug addicts / substance abusers are converted from employed status to an unemployed one.**

Increase in employment opportunities and providing employment for the treated addicts needs great care in the timing of such a help to the treated addict, believed to have been successfully de-addicted.

A treated addict remains unfit for employment for long periods subsequent to de-addiction, till such time that his de-addicted status becomes sufficiently stable and his capacity to resist Drug-

abuse compulsion, and the absence of 'Upsurges of Compulsive Urge' is sustained.

Untimely employment opportunities become counter-productive. The following factors should be kept in mind to prevent this.

a) **In order to achieve a supportive environment in the home or the workplace to which the treated addict returns, the employer as well as the family need to be fully educated about 'Drug /Substance abuse as a disease' that can re-occur (relapse).** It becomes an essential duty of the doctor, and the counsellor to impart this knowledge to the family at the time of discharge of the addict from the treating centre and during the follow-up visits.

b) The time interval between De-addiction treatment and going back to work should be decided very judiciously: the so called "De-addicted Addict" remains vulnerable to relapse as long as the "Compulsive Urge" persists.

c) A minimum period of one year is required to achieve stabilised and sustained De-addiction, that too in a supportive and 'drug-free' environment both at home and later at the place of work. Exposure of the treated addict to even a single drug/substance abuse opportunity in his home or workplace environment becomes a potential source of temptation and attraction for re-starting on drugs.

d) **The participation of the Project in-charge of the centre is very important; he / she should emphasize and repeatedly emphazise** the absolute need for the treated addict to come for frequent follow-up visits, always accompanied by the family. Contact with him should also be maintained through repeated telephonic follow-ups and get information from the family.

The relapse rate in the de-addicted addicts is alarmingly high and along with an increase in the new entrants, the drug addiction menace is becoming unmanageable. A commonly committed mistake is to terminate the indoor stay at the stage of detoxification and accept the individual as fully and completely De-addicted and fit for an early return to work. Stepping out of the house can lead to opportunities for easy availability of abuse substances. The family is unable to restrict him resulting in re-starting of drug abuse. Therefore, a De-addicted addict should be considered unemployable for a long period.

e) Complete course of de-addiction treatment, under the advice of an expert doctor, correctly timed employment, and proper support by the family, are the key factors for the recovery of the addict, which ultimately becomes an important contribution towards a reduction in the addicted population.

In this context, it is equally pertinent and important to know that a very large number of drug- addicts who are unemployed and described as (free from drug/substance-abuse) in the history sheet at the time of admission for treatment, and also those who come for consultation, gave history of starting on drugs while they were in employment (government /private service, family business, farming, self-employed). A high percentage of these unemployed drug-free at the time of history recording is of those who started on drugs **during employment / occupation.**

Observations made in the (R.C.D.A.R.C Amritsar) support the views expressed above. Analysis of the recorded histories of those addicts who were admitted for treatment and the outdoor patients from the years 2002 - 2010. In the Centre records Addicts were categorised and each category expressed as a percentage of the collective total of a number of addicts of the entire period under analysis.

a) THE UNEMPLOYED (not doing any kind of work, remaining away from the house and roaming as free wanderers)

    The highest number of addicts (36.8%) belonged to this category. An important fact is that nearly 70% of these had started on drugs while they were employed and working in some capacity or the other and became incapable of continuing their occupation as a result of starting on 'drugs'.

b) EMPLOYED:

a) **Those who gave a history of working with their family on the farm or in the family businessof these, many confessed later during counselling sessions, that they were drug-abusers (regular or periodic), and that they used isolated places in the farms for the 'addict group' meetings.**

b) Similar opportunities are available to those in service. Once out of the house, the addict can meet like minded drug users at the place of work or elsewhere at a pre-arranged meeting place. The drug-abuse remains undetected for long periods (nearly twenty-one (21.2%) percent of the total registered addicts belonged to this group).

c) Those in Government or Private service/service in the factory, employed in a hotel, stores and shops or as a transport driver. This group constituted 14.08 % of the registered addicts. The ultimate fate of these is dismissal or suspension from the job due to a decrease in their efficiency. **Addicted transport drivers remain undetected for long periods, a source of danger to themselves, passengers and others on the road.**

d) The self-employed (25.5%) is the category of those who managed their occupational work by themselves; these spend part of their earnings towards their drug abuse. They are financially independent and this supports drug-abuse which continues undetected. Ultimately the family finds out, due to their increasing inability to work and support their family. This group includes shopkeepers, daily wage earners, labourers, shoe polishers and vegetable and fruit sellers etc.

e) **PROFESSIONALS**Constitute only 0.6 % in the present analysis of the addicts'registered addicts. The very low incidence of this category is possibly due to the fact that the professionals can regulate their substance-abuse and their professional obligations without one affecting the other. These include doctors, teachers, lawyers and unskilled or skilled practitioners in other fields.

f) **STUDENTS** from school/college, graduates and post-graduate. This group formed 3.15% of the total registered addicts. (In the present Drug-abuse scenario the percentage of these at this point of time is very much higher).

Data given above makes it quite clear that in the prevalent drug addiction scenario the benefits of providing employment to the treated drug-addicts is over emphasised. Further, unemployment and lack of occupation is not the dominating contributory factor in the ever increasing number of drug-abusers.

SUMMARY

a) Those employed in Government or Private service and the self- employed and also the professionals, practitioners and students put together have time-consuming occupations and greatly outnumber the unoccupied, the unemployed the "free wanderers". It is noteworthy that in this latter category a very high percentage belonged to the employed category and lost their employment/occupation and became "free wanderers" after they started on drug abuse and ultimately became hardcore addicts.

b) The benefits of increase in job opportunities would be of limited value in improving the drug-addiction scenario because employment of imperfectly and improperly De-addicted Addicts does not help as they are prone to a very high rate of relapses; a wrongly timed occupation and employment of an imperfectly and inadequately De-addicted addict does not protect him against drug-abuse but contributes towards continuance of the drug habit. **Early return to work is an** important cause of relapses in the prevailing 'addiction' polluted environment.

c) An important facet of drug addiction is that the treated addict remains 'unemployable' for long periods, in terms of months even up to one year or more, unless he is put on a schedule of a follow-up treatment plan, inclusive of regular medical and counselling services by a psychiatry specialist, both for the treated addict and his family. This facility was available in R.C.D.A.R.C. Amritsar for those who agreed to avail of it. Dr. J.P.S. Bhatia, Doctor in-charge R.C.D.A.R.C pioneered this programme for the treated addicts.

d) In the ultimate analysis, unemployment as the cause of drug/substance-abuse (addiction) should not be over-emphasized with the family especially during counselling. It gives a wrong message for the families of addicts under treatment, without explaining further as to when their ward should be sent back to work.

To ensure that the treated addict becomes 'employable' in the correct sense, for any kind of occupation of his choice or that of the family ; the indoor de-addiction treatment schedule should be prolonged , extendable if necessary and accepted by patients and the families . Families unwilling to keep their ward in the Centre beyond one month must take the follow-up programme of Medical Care and counselling help after indoor De-addiction treatment. This provision existed in the R.C.D.A.R.C. Amritsar.

8

Religious Faith and Fervour, Worship and Prayers, And Belief in Spirituality is The Ultimate Remedy for Sustained Recovery of A Drug-Addict - It Is Not An Utopian Idea

I narrate here an incident that I witnessed in R.C.D.A.R.C. Amritsar of an addict under treatment, his aggressive behaviour due to drug abuse followed by his submissive conduct on realization of his earler wrong behaviour. The incident helped me to know his **indwelling personality and made me think deeply about it.**

- The addict was brought to my office in the Centre by a counsellor, and the addict entered visibly upset and highly irritable. He was not willing to listen to any positive suggestion either from me or from the counsellor and because as he wanted to leave for his home. In his desperate mood, he picked up a pair of big scissors from the office table and threw it at me while I was trying to convince him to stay for completing his De-addiction treatment period. Thereafter, the addict left the office in great anger. Staff on duty at the door stepped forward to stop him from going out and reprimand him. I intervened and told the staff to leave him alone. After about half an hour the addict returned to my office on his own in a very apologetic and humble manner and asked for my forgiveness. **Thereafter, he completed one month of the mandatory indoor treatment period very peacefully. He started visiting the prayer room daily.**

- The above described experience made a deep impression and confirmed my belief and also understanding that the addicts are as much human and humane when managed with proper approach.

- In the context of the above experience, my belief that every individual has an indwelling self-existent faith in the Almighty God is confirmed.

This chapter is an attempt to explain the reality of the above statement, which is normally beyond human comprehension in ordinary life.

The reality that I am attempting to put in written words is all about a self-existent, inherent faith in the Higher Supreme Power which exists in every human being. This indwelling faith and trust in the Almighty the Supreme Power, impels us to turn to Him instinctively for help in all our difficulties.

Religion is the gateway to our inner true self, controlling the inner mind and vital and guides us in our responses to the various environmental influences and habitual actions. On the basis of this firm belief, provision of a prayer room was given as much priority as the wards and offices and recreational rooms in R.C.D.A.R.C.

On the basis of the belief expressed above, drug / substance-abusers when brought by the family for admission and treatment, were put leading

questions regarding their attitude towards prayers and their belief in God and prayers. Nearly all of them stated that they believed in God and prayed regularly prior to starting on drug / substance-abuse. After starting on drug / substance-abuse, while they still believed in God inwardly, some of them stopped praying and going to a religious place because of a sense of guilt. As observed in R.C.D.A.R.C Amritsar subsequent to the first phase of treatment (detoxification), some of those who had stopped praying due to a sense of guilt resumed going to the prayer room of the Centre. Human beings pray to God seeking HIS help in a stressful situation; for recovery when suffering from any illness, for prosperity when in financial difficulty, for protection when in danger, and in many similar situations.

Interestingly on the other hand, some of the addicts confessed that they prayed to God every morning before leaving their home, for procuring 'the substance' and pleaded to him for an uninterrupted supply of the Drug. Whatever may be the nature of the demand, it shows that seeking help from God is due to an existent, in-born faith, that He helps in every kind of distress, suffering and deprivation.

We all have this implicit faith in God and while praying we also have trust that he listens to our prayers. We all know and believe in it and remember and put our demands without hesitation. That an addict does that despite his disarrayed thoughts, confirms an ever-existent faith in God in all human beings and we also believe that religious faith and regular prayers and God-dependence does not fail us in our hours of trouble.

It is of great significance that a drug addict remains shy of praying to God during his drug-abuse period and that he hesitates to go to a place of worship because of a sense of guilt as long as he is 'taking drugs'. This shows that his reverence for religious places persists despite suffering from addiction and he resumes praying when he stops using drugs. This further supports the belief that there is a self-existent relationship between each person and God.

It is not wrong to assume that the ever-existent relationship between the drug addict and his God can be awakened or re-awakened during his Deaddiction treatment. An addict under treatment needs motivational counselling towards prayers and worship, and awakening to this source of help for his recovery by his own faith in God and prayers.

The addict suffers from the disease of drug addiction affecting his mind and body. He lives a life of paradoxes and contradictions. **While he craves for the 'drug' and uses it for the pleasure it gives him,** in the deep recesses of his heart, in his deeper self, a similar craving coexists for the pleasure of freedom from the bondage/the slavery to 'drugs'. Some addicts confessed that they often prayed for this freedom in their lucid intervals between 'drug abuse' bouts.

Value of religious guidance and sustained recovery from Drug/ Substance-abuse when the addict under treatment is exposed to spiritual surroundings ,was observed in the successful De-addiction - Recovery-Rehabilitation of A.S. who began taking smack as a child, at the age of fifteen years and was treated in *R.C.D.A.R.C Amritsar. He relapsed repeatedly at short intervals. Ultimately he was taken to an

Ashram in Rishidwar. He had a remarkable recovery under the guidance of the Swami Ji of the ashram, in spite of two attempts of absconding from there. Besides him four other addicts treated in *R.C.D.A.R.C. were also sent to the same ashram after detoxification, followed by long periods of indoor De-addiction treatment. Three of them recovered and became 'drug-free' in one to two years and are now leading a normal life; one who took many years to recover, had many relapses in between and was in and out of the ashram many times. Finally, he also recovered and was rehabilitated ultimately.

The above paragraph cites the success story of addicts treated in R.C.D.A.R.C followed by aftercare in an ashram. Cases described above and similar ones not narrated here are strongly suggestive of a very positive role of religious atmosphere and spiritual guidance in the recovery of even the hardcore addicts.

In terms of Psychiatric changes, the site of 'Compulsive Urge' and repetitive use of 'drugs', its persistence and occurrence after De-addiction treatment is in the subconscious strata of the brain. Subconscious is the sub-mental base of the individual and impressions of instincts and habitual movements are stored there.

In spiritual terms, the subconscious is a subconscient strata. In humans it is the concealed consciousness of the being. This submerged part has no waking consciousness, but it receives and stores impressions which can surge up in dreams and in waking state. Possibly, these 'upsurges' are the cause of the pernicious nature of drug addiction and relapses.

When higher consciousness is established in the outer personality through prayers and spiritual understanding, this new consciousness goes down into the subconscious and changes it.

Religious fervour and worship prepare the mind, life and body. These are subordinate to the indwelling Spirit and the individual understands the meaning of spiritual refinement and there is a beginning of a spiritual character in him. In the case of addicts, this helps him to come out of the influence of the old habits submerged in the subconscious, through religious approach and self-knowledge. The concealed subconscient can be enlightened in the addict by exposure to spiritual environment and teaching during De-addiction treatment and thereafter during the recovery period.

It is when the enlightened thoughts replace those induced by drug / substance-abuse, that the behaviour, responses, reactions to surroundings and the environmental provocations are subdued and 'upsurgings' for the drug / substance-abuse gradually fade away.

Persistent enlightening of the subconscious strata through contact with the inner self by prayers and awakening of **'higher self' through spiritual teaching can weed out the submerged thoughts and feelings and perniciously persistent wrong habits.**

Medicare and Counselling is a scientifically determined external approach. It is as much necessary and its results depend upon the patience and acceptance by the addict and is further helped by perseverance of the Psychiatry expert and a supportive family. Long term medicare, counselling and follow-up visits up to minimum six months, preferably up to one year as suggested by the psychiatry experts provide further help. Non-compliance of these instructions, given at the time of discharge is one of the important causes of relapses.

I have a firm belief in the remedial value of worship, religious fervour and regular prayers if accepted by the addict under treatment and his family, for successful de-addiction.

All addicting drugs / substances act on the Limbic System, a part of the brain area involved in emotional and stressful situations. It is a region of the brain which is associated with experience of pleasure (joy) euphoria and the pleasurable experiences leaving a memory imprint which becomes the source of repetitive craving for the drug / substance–abuse as a 'compulsive urge' and a state of the persistence of addiction and drug-seeking.

As explained earlier, spiritual life can penetrate the subconscient and convert the obscurities of thought processes with increasing self-knowledge. The subconscious is thus trained and the upsurges from there are controlled. Under the influence of the higher parts of the being, old habitual responses are subdued. This is the value of providing exposure to religious environments and providing opportunity for regular worship and prayers. Thus, "Drug dependence" is replaced by "God Dependence" and helps the treated addict towards stable recovery.

9

MISCELLANEOUS (Mandatory Considerations of Practical Importance Summarised Under Selected Sub-Titles)

Environmental 'Drug-abuse' pollution due to easy availability of addicting- substances requires deft handling of the situation. **There are facets of 'the disease drug-addiction and its management' which are either not known or even if known are not given the deserved attention, or are totally overlooked. The widespread efforts aimed at de-addiction, prevention of relapses, rehabilitation of the treated addicts and decrease in the addicted population remains short of expectations. The information given hereafter is to highlight some basic factors and requirements.**

1. Detection is the responsibility of the concerned families. They should be aware of the guidelines listed hereafter.

a. There is an obvious change in the daily schedule of the addict. He is eager to go out in the morning or evening. If prevented to do so his frustration is obvious and he expresses anger even to the point of aggressive behaviour.

b. Returning home late at night, avoiding family members on return, and waking up late in the morning is a common complaint about him by the family. Gradually, the time spent at home shortens and he may even remain away from the house for days.

c. His increasing demand for money and if denied he resorts to thefts at home, of small items to begin with and even costlier ones later.

d. If the addict participates in the family business; irregularity in performance and pilferage of earnings is a common complaint of the family.

e. If the addict is a student, he becomes irregular in attendance or remains absent from the school, avoids parent-teacher meets and has poor performance in the examinations.

f. **Deteriorating 'physical' and 'mental health' and unwillingness to seek medical advice should sound a danger bell.**

    Ignorance of the family and lack of family support is a major cause of delayed detection and delay in the start of De-addiction treatment or no treatment at all.

2. Admission in a De-addiction Centre is very essential for adequate treatment.

    Most addicts are unwilling to get admitted and refuse to come to the centre even for consultation. In such cases, if the ignorant parents bring him either by force or by fraud, the addict refuses aggressively in most such cases. It is wrong to admit him in that frame of mind; he remains uncooperative and the treatment objective fails. This wrong approach by the family must be countered. Generally, the Project-in-charge herself should handle

such situations, by winning the confidence of the addict and explaining him and persuading him gently. Sometimes option of postponing admission by one / two days or more proves effective, provided he has been convinced and motivated properly.

3. Indoor De-addiction treatment restricted to ten to fifteen days as practiced in some De-addiction centres is an inadequate regime

    This result in an incomplete treatment followed by the occurrence of relapses because such a short stay achieves only Detoxification and not De-addiction. The addict, the family and friends and even some practicing doctors also appear to overlook this fact. This ignorance is most damaging, and is a major cause of relapses. Sufficiently long indoor stay is obligatory. The addict needs persuasive motivational counselling to complete the minimum period of one month as per mandatory recommendations of The Ministry Of Social Justice and Empowerment (MSJE) New Delhi / Chandigarh.

4. **Considerations during indoor treatment :**

    Very few addicts are self-motivated for admission and indoor treatment. Some get admitted after effective counselling. A large number enter unwillingly, and remain non-cooperative during the indoor stay and give all sorts of excuses for leaving the Centre. Complaints about the living facilities, food and ineffective treatment are common. If this approach does not succeed, the addict tries to abscond; any means and any route can be adopted including a threat to the staff or even man-handling. **In this context, it is necessary to know that such extreme behaviour is often due to the fact that the addict has left "his drug" at home and memory of its presence there triggers the urge to return home. In such cases, when known or suspected, the family is advised to search and destroy the addicting substance and inform their ward that they have done so.**

5. **Value of follow-up medical care and counselling treatment after discharge from the centre:**

a. Follow-up 'Medical Care' with the non-addicting substitutes and Counselling of the treated addict along with his family is absolutely necessary for stabilising De-addiction and ensuring successful recovery followed by rehabilitation. The frequency of follow-up visits and the duration for which these must be continued is planned by the Doctor-in-charge. Motivational counselling in the treating centre and cooperation by the treated addict is essential. This must be ensured by the family.

b. The families of the treated addicts who have received De-addiction treatment should accompany the treated addict for the periodic follow-up visits to the centre. This is necessary for an absolutely true picture of his conduct at home; so that timely help can be given. The family must support re-admission if it is suggested by the doctor.

6. <u>After–care at home :-</u> This literally means care of the treated addict after he has received indoor treatment and is discharged for home care. A supportive family can ensure a stable and sustained De-addiction of their ward and prevent relapses by following the guidelines given at the time of discharge. The 'Compulsive Urge' decreases gradually and eventually subsides during good after-care period at home. The risk occurrence of relapses always exists as long as 'upsurges' for the drug persist.

In the Red Cross De-addiction Centre R.C.D.A.R.C. Amritsar, Punjab, the addicts who completed one-month indoor treatment were encouraged to extend their stay with the support of their family. Some of them extended their stay up to six months. After-care through an extended stay in the treating Centre itself stabilised de-addiction more surely.

1. Existence of factors which causes relapses:

(a) Lack of family support is a major cause of delayed detection, delayed start of treatment or no treatment, and insufficient stay in the De-addiction treatment Centre, resulting in incomplete treatment and repeated recurrences.

(b) Failure on the part of the family to bring their ward to the treatment centre for regular follow-up visits and for a regular check-up.

(c) Treatment discontinued after the short detoxification period of ten to fifteen days and not followed by predetermined long term Indoor treatment with non-addicting substitutes and absence of counselling. Insufficient emphasis on precautions and instructions, both to the treated addict and his family at the time of discharge are very important factors. **Lack of awareness of the possibility of recurrence is a major cause of relapses.**

(d) Poor family aftercare, lack of observing precautions , inability to control their ward in his outgoing activities and, contact with old 'drug user friends', and ignorant handling by constant nagging and condemning the treated addict for his drug abuse, very often leads to relapses.

(e) Availability of addicting substance hidden at home by the addict before admission for indoor treatment; a very common practice by the addicts who plan to leave the Centre early. Families should search and destroy these before their ward returns home.

(f) The family allowing their ward to go back to work and start earning on the presumption that he is free of drug-urge as insisted by the treated addict himself.

2. **Early employment after treatment as a rehabilitative measure — a misconceived concept:-**

Most of the families make this mistake either due to ignorance or on account of financial compulsions; whatever may be the reason, this is the most damaging decision. Early return to work means premature exposure to provocative and tempting situations for drug/substance abuse.The addict should be considered unfit for employment for a long period after he is discharged from the Centre and the duration should be decided by the Doctor or Project Director. Thus, frequent follow-up visits and after-care assessment and counselling is essential for early remedial steps.

3. **Early marriage and expected support of the life partner to keep the De-addicted drug free:**

This is the prevailing mindset of most of the families. This is also a misconceived concept. On the contrary, marriage is not advocated earlier than one and a half to two years after successful De-addiction and recovery.

10

Conclusive Remarks-   A Supplement

I have felt the need to lay before the readers in as much brevity as possible, the conclusions and inferences drawn from my personal experience and observations and my comprehension of 'Drug addiction' as a disease and the plight of the 'individual afflicted' , the addict. This was achieved by meticulous history taking, repeated inter-active dialogues with the addicts and their families, daily follow up of each indoor patient by integrated assessment in consultation with the staff of the centre.

All this was possible with the collaboration and guidance of Dr. J.P.S. Bhatia. , Dr. in-charge psychiatry and an expert De-addiction specialist and his well-planned treatment and the follow-up programmes after discharge from the Centre introduced by him . All entries made in the Indoor patient's file and the record files were meticulously kept upto date for daily refrence.

The complimentary follow-up care by Dr. Bhatia which included medicines and counselling in his own clinic during the regular follow- up visits of the treated addicts, at short interval after discharge from the Centre, were the special features of after care in The R.C.D.A.R.C. Amritsar.

The records of indoor treatment in the Centre, counselling and related programmes were well maintained by me as the Project Incharge/Project Director cum Administrator. This is the basis of all the information in the Contemplative Compilation Manual now published as a **book**.

Data analysis primarily of telephonic follow- up of the indoor treated addicts and of follow up visits to the Centre has shown that appropriately treated addict, and given required family support during the after- care at home, remained free from 'Drug-abuse' for many years, some even up to ten years (admissions data analysis year 2000 to 2010) (Pg 138)

The families of the addicts are mostly ignorant of the nature of the damage caused by Drug addiction / substance-abuse. They do not know that Drug-addiction is a disease that takes a long time, in terms of many months, one year, and even more than that, for cure and recovery.

The essentials suggested and emphasized here in brief for result-oriented treatment and after-care are repetitions of those given in detail in the relevant preceding chapters.

An addict requires very careful and appropriate handling and persuasive motivation for indoor treatment, and a supportive attitude during the admission period and after discharge from the centre. There is a lack of this knowledge. In-depth understanding of the addict as an individual is essential. Prevalence of ignorance about the nasty grip of his 'Drug-abuse' is an important factor. **Inappropriate treatment and an inadequate short stay during indoor treatment, poor family support** at different stages and during the long recovery period, all these are always due to ignorance of the basic fundamentals for treatment / management and care. The outcome is either no recovery or a poor short-lasting one followed by relapses.

The value of public awareness programmes cannot be underestimated. Such programmes would be more effective if arranged for a few families grouped together rather than delivering the message to large gatherings. Awareness programmes for large gatherings are of limited practical value for general public at large. However, these do become beneficial for those few families who become alert to detect an addicted family member in their homes and seek medical help at the earliest possible.

In the treatment of a 'Drug-addict / Substance abuser', a personalised approach is required, to convey in detail to the addict and the family, the basic requirements for De-addiction treatment and management.

Each addict requires management with individual-specific as well as situation-specific approach for his treatment and his care thereafter. This obligatory key factor must be observed during indoor treatment and explained repeatedly if necessary, to the family at the time of the enquiry , during admission, during the indoor stay, at the time of discharge, and also during follow-up visits and also while suggesting a programme for after-care of the treated addict.

Mandatory exclusive Suggestions for the Families.

1. The addict needs proper understanding and not over indulgence by the family. **This advice is, particularly, for the mother and other family members —**

    (a) Do not consider drug abuse as a social stigma.

    (b) Do not hide the 'drug-habit' of your child once youcome to know it and notice his deteriorating health.

    (c) Good food alone is not a compensation for his health damage due to addiction. It is not enough by itself; it is more important to prevent relapses and take medical help urgently without delay (the reference to food care by the mothers is based on the history given by most of them, who believed that plenty of 'desi ghee' would prevent the health damage of their child). **In reality, it achieves only postponement and not prevention of the sad ending of a precious life.**

    (d) Many indulgent fathers also commit mistakes; their attitude swings between excessive strictness and over indulgence, the latter in the form of fulfilling all the demands of their ward 'in lieu' of his promise to leave 'drug-abuse', a promise which remains unfulfilled in most instances.

2. Caution is required if the addict insists on going home midway during indoor treatment, this may be a cunning plan to go and use the 'substance 'that he has left hidden at home for his use when he returns. **An addict is a helpless individual due to the 'Compulsive Urge' for**

the 'drug'. The family should be aware of this possibility, should search for the hidden substance and destroy it before their ward returns home from the Centre.

3. His first demand on reaching home after discharge from the centre may be the use of mobile phone, and scooter or car whichever is available, and this is accompanied by his insistence that he should be allowed to go out to meet his friends. **The family makes the most damaging mistake by fulfilling this demand.**

4. It is a folly to expect from an addict who is not sufficiently de-addicted to say no to 'drugs' ' by using his will power. **Unfortunately, an addict has neither the will nor the power. The will and the power to refuse addicting substances are the earliest casualties of 'drug-abuse' .**

5. Limitations of indoor treatment seven, ten or even up to fifteen days, merely detoxifies and does not de-addict. Will power to overcome the spurts of 'Compulsive Urge' is not restored. Detoxification is an initial step only. **It must necessarily be followed by a well planned Indoor de-addiction regime over a long period, which varies from patient to patient.** Additionally, the role of psychiatry specialist in the treatment regime is mandatory.

The ultimate aim is to ensure that de-addiction is stabilised and sustained. Inadequate, incomplete and inappropriate de-addiction is a major cause of relapses, thus increase in the number of drug-addicts continues.Unfortunately, a false satisfaction prevails that an increase in the number of de-addiction centres can reduce the addiction menace effectively. However, without appropriate treatment, regular follow-up and good after - care regime, the objective is not achieved and the addicted population continues to rise.

11

Epilogue

Some substances of vegetable origin produce a state of pleasure/joy and on account of this became habit-forming. These were discovered by mankind many centuries before Christ. These were described as habit-forming substances. Later other attributes such as, an irresistible urge to repeat their use because of their pleasure producing effect were discovered, and also the observation that when the substances were not taken, there was precipitation of physical and mental distress. This substance 'dependant' state of the individual has been **described as addiction,** subsequently specified as Drug-Addiction/Drug-Abuse/Substance-abuse.

Thus, 'pleasure' giving substances became "addictive" and the user is described as a drug-addict / substance-abuser. As the number of addicts became very large, this malady was described as a menace. Presently, when it has acquired unmanageable dimensionsit is a threatening epidemical disease which is spreading very fast, especially amongst the young population by now victimising the school children as well, even of the age of seven to eight years.

The remedial measures to stall the spread of drug-addiction have not proved effective enough, and the number of addicts continues to increase by geometrical progression. Ministry of Social Justice and Empowerment (M.S.J.E) New Delhi / Chandigarh sponsors De-addiction-cum-Rehabilitation programmes run by the Red Cross and NGOs through the sanction of Grant for this project. In the past few years, a large number of Government and private De-addiction Centres have come into existence, yet the rise in the number of drug-addicts continues. The universally accepted reason for this has been, the rampant availability of addicting substances/drugs to the addicts, and each day an increasing number of individuals are lured to join the existing groups.

While the availability of abuse substances remains the major undeniable fact, it should not be allowed to overshadow an equally important factor responsible for the unchecked rise in the addicted population. There is re-occurrence of addiction (relapse) sooner or later in a large number of drug-addicts who are supposedly de-addicted in a De-addiction Centre.

The major cause of occurrence of relapse in spite of indoor De-addiction treatment is "the poverty of knowledge and understanding of drug / substance - abuse and its victim the Addict and, inadequate / incomplete treatment because of the following reasons".

(A) Short duration of indoor stay without proper follow-up programme and a faulty after - care.

(B) Absence of fool-proof measures against the entry of addicting substances into the De-addiction Treatment Centres.

(C) Lack of adequate and effective counselling during Indoor De-addiction treatment.

(D) Insufficient counselling of the family during the indoor stay and at the time of discharge from the Centre and at the time of repeated follow-up visits.

(E) **Lack of rapport between the staff and the addict under indoor treatment; this rapport forms the basis of individual-specific relationship with the addict and building up his confidence in the treatment during his stay in the centre.**

An addict needs a comprehensive approach during the medical treatment of addiction; the Doctor In-charge should be a psychiatry specialist to detect and treat any concurrent Psychiatric changes in his behaviour, pre-existing or precipitated due to drug/substance - abuse.

The essentials for recovery after De-addiction treatment are (a concise repetition of what has been given in detail in various chapters):

1. Early detection of the drug-addiction problem in a family member. A vigilant family, aware of its possibility in the prevailing scenario of drug-addiction, must always remain alert and vigilant.

2. **Acceptance by the family that addiction is a treatable disease and not a social stigma; the drug user will not be able to reject 'drug' on his own and he requires indoor treatment in a De-addiction cum Rehabilitation Centre.**

3. Once the addict is admitted, the family should be educated through repeated counselling, to give full moral support during indoor treatment, and also motivate him to complete the period of indoor stay as advised by the doctor.

4. During indoor treatment, the family cooperation with the administration of the Centre against the availability of any kind of addicting substances, including tobacco, is an important aspect of the required family support.

5. **During the indoor stay, a comprehensive approach in the Medical Care by the Doctor in-charge, regular counselling by the Counsellor, regular interactive dialogue with the addict and his family by the Project in-charge, who should also ensure maintenance of a confidence-inspiring atmosphere in the Centre to promote a positive attitude in the addict under treatment; all these are the pre-requisites for proper recovery.**

6. **Provision of additional services such as :**

   a. Occupational therapy with minor handcraft facilities which helps the addict under treatment to remain free of repeatedly occurring thoughts centred on old memories of drug/substance-abuse and its joy / pleasure .

   b. Facilities for physical exercise and indoor games.

   c. **A prayer room and availability of religious books for individuals and group meetings.**

7. **Good nourishing diet according to a diet schedule which should be displayed prominently for the notice of the inmates and their families.**

8. **At the time of discharge of the treated addict, family should be counselled including advice on follow-up care while he is in the care of the**

family at home ; this being a crucial period for good recovery.

i) The family has to ensure that he does not re-establish any contact with his old substance-abuser friends (his peer group); also that he does not leave the house unescorted.

ii) He should not have any access to money.

iii) He should not be allowed to keep a mobile with him and he should not be permitted to use any transport belonging to him or the family.

9. **Recovery at home is also the joint responsibility of the family and the Treatment Centre** to give continued help in keeping the treated addict drug-free after he is discharged from the Centre.

10. The Centre must encourage the family to bring him for regular follow up visits for counselling and medicinal treatment if necessary; the occurrence of relapse must be detected early for re-admission at the earliest.

11. There is yet another important joint responsibility of the Centre and the family. It is based on the concept of exposure to religious teachings and motivation for prayers, for building up positive thinking, and increasing will power of the treated addict to reject 'drug' offers and suppress upsurges of 'Compulsive Urge'.

12. **For the treated addict to be properly de-addicted a sufficiently long period of at least one year is required after discharge from the**

Centre. This period may be spent at his own home, or in an after-care home. A substitute for these is an extended stay in the treatment Centre. The aim is to prevent exposure to any tempting circumstances. During this period he should not be allowed to handle money, mobile and household transport. It helps towards sustained De-addiction and a stable Rehabilitation when he goes back to work.

This Book, based on personal experience gained from the management of The Red Cross De-addiction Centre, Amritsar, contains all the helpful details for providing maximum opportunity for good after-care and recovery through near-ideal even if not the absolutely ideal atmosphere, for general and medical care in a treating Centre.

I had the providential good fortune of having been a Pharmacology teacher for twenty-six years in Medical College, Amritsar and teaching on addicting substances, addiction and treatment of addiction. After retirement in the year 1987, I had the God-ordained opportunity to learn about Drug addiction/Substance abuse from the patients themselves. I acknowledge most humbly that I knew little about the various practical aspects of the subject of Drug-addiction/Substance-abuse required to be known for practical management of a De-addiction cum Rehabilitation Centre and the addicts admitted for treatment. In this respect, the Pharmacology Text Book did not provide the required contents, and in the limited hours for the teaching of these chapters, I could impart only the 'Book Knowledge' to the future doctors treating addicts in their clinical practice. This Book by me, if taken seriously by them, can provide useful reference source for upgrading their approach in their clinical practice.

My effort was to keep the team in The Treatment Centre woven together sharing a common motto of 'service before self' and move on with patience towards a common aim of giving good care for a good recovery. Dr. Bhatia, the doctor in-charge, Smt. Dalbir Kaur, the nurse, and I joined The R.C.D.A.R.C Amritsar on its inauguration day in October 1995, and we all worked together till its closure in 2010/11.

An appeal to the medical practitioners, on behalf of the victims of drug-addiction ; because drug-addiction is rampant and is out of proportion to the availability of De-addiction Centres . Therefore, treatment of Drug-addicts has also become a part of general medical practice with most of the medical practitioners. It is obligatory for them to have **knowledge of Drug - addiction / Substance-abuse as a disease** which requires prolonged after-care besides the use of De-addicting drugs (non-addicting substitutes).

A long term follow-up and aftercare is indispensable for sound recovery rehabilitation and joining the mainstream of life.

The life journey of a Drug/Substance-abuser is full of difficulties for himself and his family. Problems of his addicted state are not fully appreciated and his De-addiction treatment is beset with medical challenges.

I end with gratitude for the opportunity that came in my way for this section of the population because their disease is mostly poorly understood by all those who treat them and plan for their welfare.

Even as good efforts were put in by **The Red Cross De-addiction-cum-Rehabilitation Centre (R.C.D.A.R.C.) Amritsar** and its staff; all efforts must come to an end sometimes and pave the way for even better which should follow hopefully.

Addendum 1

From: - Dr. Mrs. Saroje Sanan

The few pages that follow in Hindi have been written by me to express the feelings and sentiments of the addicts under treatment, shared with me by them. These are written primarily in the form of poetry and partly as prose wherever necessary.

नशावान / नशा ग्रस्त की दुर्गम जीवन यात्रा का आंरभ और समस्त जीवन की कठिनाइयों की व्याख्या

मां की आचल से निकला तो जा गिरा नशे की निर्दई गोद में । नशे की आलिंगन में था मां का प्यार और जिंदगी की अनेक बहारें । उसके पश्चात नशा लेना और नशे में डूबे रहना बन गई जीवन के हर पल की कठोर आवश्यकता और विवशता ।

नशा केवल अभिशाप नही एक अनोखा रोग है। नशा करने वाला परिस्थितियों का शिकार है। जिस समाज और परिवार की अज्ञानता की यह देन नशावान को मिली है , उसी समाज और परिवार का कर्तव्य है कि वह उसे नशा मुक्त करने में पूरा सहयोग दें।

नशा एक भयानक रोग है और अब तक एक महामारी का रूप क्यों ले चुका है ? इसका इलाज क्यों एक चुनौती बन गया है ? नशा करने वाला व्यक्ति नशीले पदार्थ लिए बिना नहीं रह सकता। शारीरिक और मानसिक स्तर पर नशे का बंदी बन जाता है। नशा लेना उसका शौक नही , विवशता है। यह कड़वा सत्य मानकर और समझकर ही

परिवार को तथा इलाज करने वालों को नशावान की पूर्ण सहायता करनी आवश्यक है।

साधारणतया, नशावान नशा थोड़ी मात्रा में शुरू करता है। धीरे-धीरे या तेजी से यह मात्रा बढ़कर कई गुना हो जाती है। नशा न लेने से उसे अत्यंत शारीरिक कष्ट होता है। उसके साथ ही अत्यंत मानसिक तनाव और बेचैनी भी होती है । नशा लेना ही जीवन का एकमात्र उद्देश्य तथा उसको प्राप्त करना ही उसकी दिनचर्या का लक्ष्य बन जाता है।

परिवार के साथ दिन रात का संघर्ष भरा संबंध, और नशा हमसफरो के साथ अपनापन और अटूट मेलजोल हर नशावान की जीवन गाथा बन जाती है। मां-बाप, भाई-बहन, पत्नी और बच्चों के लिए कोई सोच नहीं रहती। इन सब के प्रति स्नेह भी नशे की धुंधली सोच में आलोप हो जाता है।

पढ़ाई में अरुचि हो जाती है और व्यवसाय के लिए अक्षमता और उसमें असफलता। नशे की प्राप्ति के लिए धन का दुरुपयोग , घर में चोरी , झगड़ा , धमकियां देना नशेवान का व्यावहारिक स्वभाव बन जाता है। जब धन की पूर्ति घर से नहीं होती तब नशेवान जुर्म की दुनिया में प्रवेश करता है। लूटमार, चोरी, और मारपीट दिनचर्या का दुखदाई अंश बन जाता है।

ऊपर संक्षेप में हैं नशा और उसके असीमित असर।

नशेवान की जीवन शैली उसके परिवार के लिए असहनीय परिस्थिति बन कर सारे परिवार को विनाश की ओर ले जाती है। विनाश से बचाने के लिए और नशेवान को नशा मुक्त करने में पूर्ण इलाज की आवश्यकता है। दुर्भाग्य है कि यह परिस्थितियां पैदा हुई हैं और जंगल में लगी आग की तरह बढ़ रही हैं । आग बढ़ती जा रही है और इसको रोकने के लिए समय हाथ से निकला जा रहा है। देश

की युवा शक्ति विलीन हो रही है। गंभीर स्तिथि हमें विवश करती है कि हम इसको ओर आगे बढ़ने से रोकने के लिए संबंधित प्रशनों का का उत्तर ढूंढे और समाधान निकाले। प्रबंधकों का सहयोग अत्यंत आवश्यक है।

हम सबको क्या करना चाहिए , क्या कर सकते हैं और किस तरह सफलता पा सकते है यही सोच है मेरी दिन रात की , और आकांक्षा है आपके सहयोग की।

नशा संबंधित प्रशन :-

++

- नशा क्या है-- किस प्रकार का रोग है ?

- कैसे आरंभ होता है, उसके लक्षण क्या है ?

- नशावान के व्यक्तित्व में क्या परिवर्तन आते हैं ?

- नशेवान की निजी जीवन पर, परिवार पर और समाज पर क्या प्रभाव है ?

- नशा कितने प्रकार के हैं ? नशा एक महामारी की तरह क्यों फैल रहा है ? इसको रोकने में विवशता क्यों है ?

- वर्तमान परिस्थिति में परिवार क्या कर सकता है.....समाज का क्या सहयोग हो सकता है.....प्रशासन अपने उपाय को और अधिक सफल कैसे बना सकता है ?

- नशेवान के शुभचिंतक उसके इलाज के प्रति कितने कर्तव्यशील हो सकते हैं! ++

++ उपर लिखे "प्रसंग" में मेरे अनुभव और सोच के अनुसार इन सब प्रशनो के उत्तर पुस्तक के अंग्रेजी के भिन्न-भिन्न भागों में कथित है!++

नशा करने वालों के व्यक्तित्व को पूर्ण गहराई से समझने के लिए तथा केवल नशा रहित ही नही बल्कि नशा मुक्त बनाने के लिए किस सोच की आवश्यकता है ?

इस पुस्तक की लेखिका की ओर से एक नशावान की जीवन गाथा , उसकी दर्द भरी पुकार , जीवन की हर पहलू में उसकी विवशता और उसकी व्यवस्था । नशावान के व्यक्तित्व में आए बदलाव ओर उसके कारण, और उसको नशा मुक्त करने में सबकी ओर से क्या क्या उपाय किए जा सकते है। **नशावान कैसे अनुभव करता है और उसका समाधान चाहता है मैने एक कविता के रूप में लिखा है।**

प्रस्तुत है एक नशा-ग्रस्त की पुकार -----

मेरे शुभचिंतको सुनो मेरी उलझनों भरी जीवन गाथा !!

मैं कोई ऐसी पहेली नहीं जिसे आप सुलझा ना सको,
यही मान कर और समझ कर ही मुझे अपना लो ।

मैं हूं ऐसे एक भंयकर अनोखे रोग का लाचार शिकार ,
अदृश्य जंजीरों से बधां हुआ हूं मैं और मेरा व्यवहार।

मेरा जीवन असंगत विचारों की श्रृंखला बन गया है ,
जीवन आशा निराशा की अटूट लड़िया बन गया है ।

मेरा जीवन लंबी कहानी है बार बार हार और जीत की ,
मेरा जीवन है अंधेरी गलीयों से उभरी भ्रष्ट सोच की ।

इस उभरती दुहार का बंधी मैं लाचार, इसे ठुकरा नहीं सकता,
इस उभरती हुंकार के अधीन लाचार, इसे भुला नहीं सकता ।

मेरे शुभ चिंतको, मित्रो, समाज के रखवालो और परिजनो,
मुझे बचाने के लिए , धैर्य और ज्ञान से समझो और जानो।

क्यों लेता हूं नशा बार बार, होश में आता हूं तो प्रण करता हूं ,
सोच की अंधेरी गलियों से पुकार आती है तो चल पढ़ता हूं।

अपने परम साथी को ढूंढने और उससे लिपटने के लिए ,
यह ही बन जाती है दिनचर्या एक भरपूर जीवन के लिए।

जेब भरी हो तो अपने प्रिय की खोज में निकल पड़ता हूं ,
मिले तो नापता ऊंचाई पहाड़ो की, बिछड़े तो गिड़गिड़ाता हूं।

मेरे चिकित्सक और स्वास्थ्य के रखवालो , सुनो मेरी पुकार,
आपके पूर्ण ज्ञान से हो सकता है मेरा छुटकारा और सुधार ।

अनगिनत नशा छुड़ाओ केंद्र हैं हम नशावानो के इलाज के लिए,
दस बीस दिन का इलाज करते हैं, नशे से मुक्त करने के लिए।

नशामुक्त करने का दावा तो सब करते हैं , छुपा दबंग देख पाते नहीं ,
इलाज से अस्थाई नशा रहित हो जाते हैं, पर नशा मुक्त होते नहीं ।

ना छोड़ो हमें अधूरे इलाज की नाज़ुक दशा में बीच मंझदार,
बार बार उभरती रहती है अंदर से नशे की हुंकार और पुकार ।

मेरे चिकित्सको , शुभचिंतको , मैं हूं इस रोग से बेबस और लाचार,
तुम तो ज्ञान के सागर हो , ना छोड़ो मुझे इस तरह से बीच मंझदार ।

आशा निराशा की जुगल बंदी से मुक्त किए बिना घर भेज देते हो,
मैं तो नादान हूं , लाचार हूं , तुम तो नशा-रोग के महान विशेषज्ञ हो ।

नशा मुक्त हुए बिना, सौंप देते हो परिजनों की देख रेख के लिए,
परिजन प्रसन्न होकर हमें बाहर भेज देते हैं धन कमाने के लिए।

परिवार करता है हम पर भरोसा, और मित्र हमारी सरहाना करते हैं ,
हम एक अस्थाई जीत पर, प्रसन्नता की तरंगो में झूमते खो जाते हैं ।

परिवार के भरोसे से मिली स्वतंत्रता और हमारा नया आत्मविश्वास ,
बढ़ते कदम हमें ले चलते है बार बार पुराने नशावान मित्रों के पास।

फिर हुए गुमराह पुराने हमसफरों के साथ हम बेखबर घूमते रहे ,
फिर से गुमराह हुए कोई रोक न सका, नशा पदार्थ मिलते रहे ।

इस तरह नवजीवन की आशा और सुखद सपने बिखर जाते हैं,
सोच की अंधेरी गलियों से उभरी पुकार , तो जुड़े नाते टूट जाते हैं ।

असफलता से , अज्ञानता से लाचार फिर से सहता हूं दुत्कार ,
रोक न सका अपने आप को फिर बन गया मैं बड़ा गुनहगार ।

मुझे प्यार दुलार चाहिए , मुझ लाचार को अपने सीने से लगाओ ,
नशा-मुक्त इलाज केंद्र में बहुत दिन ठहराओ, भरपूर समझाओ ।

सफल नशा मुक्त जीवन को सशक्त बनाना निर्भर आप पर,
घर आने पश्चात हम क्या करते हैं, परिवार होता है बेखबर।

निश्चिंत परिवार भरोसा कर , बाहर जाने को नही करता इंकार ,
रात नशा ग्रसत हो कर लौटने पर , छुपा लेता है मां का दुलार।

केंद्र के " काउंसलर " घर पहुंचते हैं हमारी दशा जानने के लिए ,
बाहर हमसफरों के साथ हैं , बताती नहीं मां हमें बचाने के लिए ।

यह परिणाम है " होम विसिटस " और उन पर निर्भर रिकॉर्ड का ,
अमृतसर स्थित नशा छुड़ाओ केंद्र ने किया बहिष्कार इस क्रिया का।

केवल केंद्र में " फौलो अप विज़िटस" से ही होता है ठीक अनुमान,
"विज़िटस " में परिवार सहित आए नशा मुक्त की ठीक पहचान ।

केंद्र के संचालको , नशा मुक्ती के लिए मुझे परिवार सहित बुलाओ,
मेरे परिजनो और शुभचिंतको, मेरी इस आवश्यकता को न भुलाओ।

मेरे चिकित्सको मुझे सशक्त बनाओ , नशा मुक्त रहूं स्वयं इच्छा से , प्रभावित ना हो जाऊं नशा उपलब्ध केप्रलोभन और आंधियों से ।

मेरे शुभचिंतको , मेरे चिकित्सको , नशा छुड़ाओ केंद्रों के प्रबंधको और संचालको , हम नशावानो की सोच के नीचे लिखे उदाहरण पढ़िए। मेरे नशा ग्रस्त जीवन के दो सत्य नीचे लिखित स्वयं-सूचना में हैं।

नशावानों की ओर से :-

जागरूकता के ज्ञान भरे भाषणों से हमे शिक्षा प्रदान करते हो , नशा विरुद्ध अनगिनत रैलियों का प्रबंध भी कई बार करते हो ।

जानकर आश्चर्य होगा, मैं तो वहां स्वयं इच्छा से ही जाता हूं , वहां पुराने साथियों को मिलकर अंदर ही अंदर मुस्कुराता हूं।

हमसफर नहीं मिलते है तो बेगानो को ही अपना बना लेता हूं , नशा करके जाता हूं , जोश में नशा विरुद्ध दौड़ों में भागता हूं।

कोई नही जान सकता कि जेब में हम नशा पदार्थ लेकर जाते हैं , जीभ नीचे या शरीर के अदृश्य हिस्सों में नशा भंडार छुपाते हैं।

नही समझोगे कितने दिलेर हैं हम नशा पदार्थ बांटने के लिए , हर अवसर ढूढते हें हमसफरों को इशारों से बताने के लिए।

नशे के अधीन हैं हम , और नशेवानों से है हमें असीमित प्यार , नशा ग्रसत रहना हमारा जीवन , नशावान हमसफर परिवार ।

केंद्र को नाम देते हैं नशा मुक्त और मुड़ बसेरा। घर भेजने के लिए विचार करो गंभीरता से। तन की पिड़ा से मुक्त होना नशा मुक्ती नही होती। अधूरे इलाज से नशा मुक्ती की आशा अज्ञानता है। इस तरह हम और हमारा परिवार विश्वास खौ देते है।

बड़े जलसो में जागरूक किया , शपथ दिलवाई और हमने प्रण लिए,
आपका कर्तव्य हो गया , हमें गहराई में समझे बिना आप चल दिए।

नुक्कड़ नाटकों में शराबी दिखाया हंसते दर्शको ने किया तिरस्कार ,
हमें क्या मिला , ना हमदर्दी , ना नशे से छूटकारा इलाज का उपहार ।

मुझें तो सब नशावान बुलाते है और भी हैं संसार में नशे के शिकार
नशा कुर्सी का, धन बटोरने का , और भी हैं अनेको नशे के प्रकार ।

नशा उपलब्ध करवाने वाले गुनहगारों का शिकार मैं बन गया हूं ।
इस प्रचलित सत्य को सब तो जानते है फिर में ही बदनाम क्यों ।

**नशा मुक्ति के सफल इलाज के लिए एक अनमोल सोच और
दृष्टिकोण की व्याख्या.....**

भगवान पर विशवास हमारी संस्कृति में अमूल्य माना जाता है। इस
भावना के अधीन आर.सी.डी.ऐ.आर.सी. अमृतसर , में दाखिल हुए
नशावानो को प्राथना के कमरे में जाने के लिए उत्साहित करना केंद्र
का एक अहम यत्न था और इसके लिए योगा चिकित्सक उत्साहित
करते थे । कुछ नशावान पूजा के कमरे में स्वयं प्रेरणा से जाते थे।कुछ
को समझा बुझा कर ले जाना पड़ता था । इसके प्रसंग में दो मूल्यवान
उदाहरण दिए जाते है :-

1.) एक नशावान ने बताया कि गुरुद्वारे जाने की उसकी अटूट
दिनचर्या बचपन से ही रही है । परंतु नशा-सेवनकी आदत पढ़ जाने
के बाद इस दिनचर्या को नही निभाया क्योंकि वो नशा करने के
पश्चात गुरुद्वारा जाना भगवानका अपमान समझता था। इसी केंद्र में
रहते हुए नशा रहित होने के पश्चात वह पूजा के कमरे में रोज जाने
लगा और इसी केंद्र में नशा मुक्ति के पश्चात एक अनुभवी कोंसलर
के पद पर लगभग एक साल योगदान दिया।

2.) कुछ दाखिल हुए नशावानो ने बताया कि वो भी भगवान पर भरोसा करते थे । घर से नशा लेने के लिए बाहर जाने से पहले हर बार अपने पूज्य भगवान को याद करते और उस से विनम्र प्राथना करते थे कि नशा उपलब्ध करवाने में हमारी अचूक सहायता करें।

यह दो उदाहरण बताने का तात्पर्य है कि इनसे एक स्पष्ट संदेश मिलता है। हर व्यक्ति के अंदर न मिटने वाला भगवान के प्रति प्रेम भी है और विश्वास भी स्थापित है ।

किसी भी नशा छुड़ाओ केंद्र में इस अंतर्गत स्थित विश्वास को उजागर करना नशे के इलाज में प्रयोग किया जासकता है , किया जाना चाहिए। प्रार्थना और अध्यात्मिकता के इस प्रयोग के विषय में मेरी इस पुस्तक में एक पूरा अध्याय है। उस अध्याय के आधार पर में एक सुझाव आपके सामने नतमस्तक होकर लिखती हूं।

नशा छुड़ाओ केंद्रो में धार्मिक वातावरण , धार्मिक भजनों , गुरबाणी और धार्मिक संगीत नाद के स्पंदन नशारहित / नशा मुक्त इलाज का सबसे अधिक सफल प्रयास हो सकता है। यह मेरा अटूट विश्वास है। इसलिए मेरा सुझाव है कि इस क्रिया को हर नशा छुड़ाओ केंद्र को अपनाना चाहिए ।

भगवान की पूजा की लगन का उजागर होना और भगवान की शक्ति के आगे नशा लगाव को समर्पित करने से नशावान का नशे के प्रति झुकाव के स्थान पर अध्यात्मिक सोच का प्रभूत्व उजागर हो सकता है । **मैं इस विश्वासके साथ नशा छुड़ाओ केंद्रो के संचालको से प्रार्थना करती हूं और आग्रह भी कि इस विचार धारा को केंद्रो में क्रियाशील किया जाए।**

लेखक :- डॉक्टर सरोज सानन

The Red Cross De-Addiction-cum-Rehabilitation Centre (R.C.D.A.R.C.) Amritsar, Punjab. India

This Centre was initially established as a De-addiction Centre by the Indian Red Cross society, District Branch Amritsar, and I was appointed as Project Co-ordinator to manage the same. Subsequently, over the years the Centre was upgraded to...The Red Cross De-addiction-cum-Rehabilitation Centre (R.C.D.A.R.C.).

The Centre came into existence with the far-sighted vision of the Chair Person Mrs. Poonam Sidhu (Assistant Commissioner ITS). It was inaugurated after an awareness program on Drug /Substance-abuse (drug-addiction) presided by the Deputy Commissioner Mr. Karan Bir Sidhu (IAS.) accompanied by the Chair Person Mrs. Poonam Sidhu (ITS), in the village Ghanupur Distt. Amritsar; this village was reported to have a very large number of 'drug-addicts'. Subsequent to meeting the addicts and their families decision was taken to start a De-addiction Centre for admission and treatment of the addicts on the first floor of The Red Cross Sarai situated within the premises of Guru Nanak Dev Hospital, Majitha Road, Amritsar.

A simple inauguration of Red Cross De-addiction Centre took place on 2-10-1995 and the first batch of ten Drug-addicts/ Substance-abusers of the village Ghanupur was admitted on 3-10-1995 for indoor De-addiction treatment for ten days as decided by the Red Cross Chair Person ; duration of treatment was in accordance to the practice followed by other De-addiction Centres.

Subsequently, the duration of indoor De-addiction treatment and the management norms for the Centre were improved upon progressively over the years to give the best possible care to the addicts. This was possible with the unstinted support of the Chair Person Mrs. Sidhu at whose behest this Centre was started. The Centre functioned successfully for more than fifteen years from the year 1995 to early 2011.During this period more than two thousand seven hundred addicts were treated as indoor patients and nearly seven thousand attended the outpatient for enquiry for the new patients, after – care treatment and follow-up visits.

The aim and the objective of this Centre was to provide the best possible Medical Care and general care during admission in the Centre. All of us serving in the Centre tried our best to achieve the same.

The MOTTO "SERVICE BEFORE SELF "was the guiding principle in the functioning of R.C.D.A.R.C. it was accepted and practiced in letter and spirit. This was possible with the examples set by the Dr.- in –charge, the Project Director, the Manager and the Counsellors. This ideology and its supportive atmosphere in the Centre was maintained throughout the period of its growth from a De-addiction Centre (R.C.D.A.C) to a De-addiction - cum Rehabilitation Centre R.C.D.A.R.C. The whole staff of the Centre put in their best possible efforts in the routine management and dealings, as well as in the frequent challenging situations created individually or collectively by 'the addicts under treatment'.

MANAGEMENT DETAILS :-

Staff appointments: The Doctor, Project - Coordinator, Administrator, Counsellor and Nurse were appointed prior to the inauguration of the Red Cross De-addiction Centre.

Duties performed by the staff :

1 **The Doctor In-charge:** Dr. J. P. S. Bhatia M. D. (Psychiatry with "Drug - Addiction" as the subject of his thesis). Dr. Bhatia offered to work without any emoluments, and continued to do so through out the period of fifteen years that the Centre functioned; except for the period (Sept I999 to 2003) ; when he was given a salary from the sanctioned Project Grant-in-aid.

(a) Assessment of each addict before admission. (b) Initial **detoxification** treatment followed by **the De-addiction regime**. (c) Daily visits to the Centre and recording of daily progress in the case files. (d) **Planning of follow-up and after-care programmes subsequent to indoor treatment.**

Medical Care: The medicines prescribed by the doctor were all purchased by the Centre. Besides the specific de-addicting medicines and those required for any concurrent illness formed a part of the medical care provided by the Centre.

Basic laboratory investigations were done for every addict who was to be admitted. The report of the investigations was checked by the Doctor-in-charge prior to admission of the addict. An addict requiring opinion of a specialist for a concurrent illness was also provided this facility. All expenses were met with by the Centre. **The Centre practiced a holistic approach in the De-addiction treatment of an addict; this was always considered of paramount importance above any kind of financial considerations.**

2. **Project Co-ordinator subsequently promoted to Project Director :-**

    Dr. Mrs. Saroje Sanan M.B.B.S. (Dlh) Ph.D. (Edin.UK). Former Professor and Head of The Pharmacology Department Government Medical College, Amritsar was initially appointed as Project Co-ordinator.In the year 1997, the post of manager/administrator was abolished due to paucity of funds and the Project co-ordinator offered to perform additional duties of the above administrator. Later in 1999 the Ministry of Social Justice and Empowerment (M.S.J.E) New Delhi, sanctioned grant for the Centre and designated Project Co-ordinator as Project-Director. She worked without accepting emoluments from the year 1995 to2010/11 when the Centre was closed. Any emoluments given to her were donated back as such regularly to the R.C. office and copies of the written records of the same were maintained in the Centre.

In November 1995, The Project Co-ordinator was asked by the Chairperson Red Cross society to collect donations for the De-addiction Centre because of the financial difficulties faced by The Red Cross office. **The treatment of the addicts in the Centre was to be free of any charges**. Dr. Sanan as Project Co-ordinator, offered to collect donations on behalf of the Red Cross office. More than one lakh rupees were collected in the first month. Collection of donations by her continued as long as the Centre remained functioning however, the donated amounts decreased gradually over the years. **A complete record of the collected donations was maintained by her and the office was kept informed in writing regularly by the Project Co-ordinator later promoted to Project Director, throughout the period R.C.D.A.R.C. remained functional.**

Duties Performed by the Project Co-ordinator / Projector Director-cum-administrator :

1.) Personal presence of the Project Director at the reception desk along with the counsellor and the nurse, to ensure a cordial, confidence inspiring atmosphere at the time of first exposure of the addict and the family to the Centre, so that the addicts were adequately motivated for indoor De-addiction treatment. 2.) **Training of the ward staff and the other helpers to create a positive atmosphere for the management of the Centre and for an ethical behaviour and proper dealings with the**

admitted addicts. 3.) To ensure that instructions by the Doctor in-charge for the admitted addicts, are meticulously followed by the nurse on duty. 4.) Oversee that the Medical Care prescribed by the doctor was properly carried out by the nurse and its entries made in the case files regularly. 5.) **Uninterrupted availability of the medicines prescribed by the doctor.** 6.) Ensuring clean and healthy living conditions for the admitted addicts. 7.) Providing palatable and nourishing diet for the addicts **(The daily diet chart was displayed prominently for the inmates to know and make a demand for its fulfilment if so needed).** 8.) **Take effective steps for guarding against the entry of addicting substances, unwanted intruders in the garb of relatives, friends and strangers, through strict checking arranged at the entrance door.** 9.) Measures for preventing absconding of the admitted addicts (all windows sealed with wire gauze and glass doors with grills in between . 10.) Maintenance of accounts and official correspondence with The Red Cross office (there was no sanctioned clerical post in the Centre).

Collection of donations by the Project co-ordinator / Director-cum-Administrator continued due to the following compulsions and circumstances:

A) Long delays in receiving the sanctioned funds. B) Low monthly emoluments of the employed staff in the sanctioned grant and their dissatisfaction. This necessitated supplementation from the collected donations to avoid financial dissatisfaction of the staff which could affect the services to the admitted addicts. C) **For payment** of salaries to the extra staff for improvement services in the Centre - (i) Cook for in-house cooked food for the inmates. (ii) For Occupational Therapy and training of minor handcraft to the addicts. (iii) Computer coaching. (iv) Provision of facilities for Indoor games.

3. The Manager: Mr. R.K. Kapoor was appointed on this post from 1995 to 1996 and was followed by appointment of a retired Colonel for the year 1997. Thereafter, the post was abolished by the then President Red Cross Society District Branch, Amritsar, and the Project- Co-ordinator was asked to take up the additional charge.

4. The Counsellors: Miss Prarthana, (M.A. Psychology), was appointed. She started with the first batch of the admitted addicts and continued till the year 1997. Thereafter Miss Kulwinder Kaur, (M.A. Psychology), took over and stayed on the post till the year 2002. **Subsequently, regular counsellors could not be appointed because of the low salaries offered to them.** Thenceforth, addicts treated in the Centre and those who remained drug-free for one year or more and were kept under observation in the Centre or with follow up visits, were appointed as Experimental Counsellors (designation recognised by The Ministry of Social Justice and Empowerment (M.S.J.E.) New Delhi. Four such counsellors worked between the year 2002 and 2010/11.

The Counsellors recorded detailed preliminary history of each addict who came to the Centre for consultation /admission and treatment

(a) Those who came to the Centre for enquiry were given motivational counselling for indoor De-addiction treatment. (b) The admitted addicts were counselled individually alone, as well as along with the family. (c) Separate family counselling sessions were scheduled to educate the family about the necessity of full support during indoor treatment. (d) Frequent group sessions were held to make the addicts aware of addiction as a disease and causes of relapse after treatment. (e) Addicts were encouraged sharing between themselves and for mutual help to complete the full course of De-addiction treatment.

5. The Nurse: Smt. Dalbir Kaur was appointed in 1995 starting her duties with the first admitted batch of addicts. She had the experience of nursing in a private hospital. A very willing and disciplined worker who worked tirelessly, putting in extra hours of duty without any demand for extra benefits. Her dealing with the patients was correct and she remained an asset for the Centre till the closure of the Centre.

6. The Ward Boys: Four attendants were appointed by the Red Cross Office initially. Two worked as ward boys on night duty, one as gatekeeper and one for general duties. When three of these left, the vacancies were not filled by R.C. office on account of lack of funds.

Later, in order to maintain satisfactory care of the patients and their safety at night, two ward boys were appointed with the permission of the R.C. office. The salary payment was arranged from the donations collected on behalf of the

R. C. office. This was an absolutely essential step because the addicts undergoing the initial phase of treatment (Detoxification) suffer from severe withdrawal distress and are very restless and require appropriate care. Sh. Gurcharan Singh 'Babbi' was appointed as the senior night ward boy in the year 2003, and he stayed till the year 2010/11 when the Centre was closed. **He proved to be a very efficient night ward boy and could manage all the challenging situations efficiently.**

7. The Gatekeeper : A full-time gatekeeper was necessary for guarding the entrance of the Centre. Initially, one of the attendants worked as the gatekeeper in addition to his general duties. The arrangement was satisfactory as long as the Centre accommodation was confined to the first floor of the Red Cross Sarai. Later with the growth of the Centre in terms of services, activities of the inmates, provision for indoor games and cooking arrangements in the Centre, **and expansion of accommodation to the ground floor**, the appointment of a regular day time gatekeeper/guard was necessary. Sh. Satpal Sharma, a retired IPS. Sipahi was appointed and his duties at the entrance included: (a) to ensure that the entrance door remained closed except when the entry of any person was to be allowed as decided by the administrator. (b) A thorough physical checking of 'the addict' and the accompanying family was done before they were allowed to approach the reception area. (c) To retain and check belongings brought by them, and allowing only the permitted items when the addict was admitted for indoor treatment.

(d) **Most importantly, strict checking was done for money in cash and otherwise, jewellery on a person or in the belongings and, personal wrist watch, mobile etc.** (e) Knives or scissors or other sharp-edged items, nail cutters, mirrors, steel spoons and any other suspicious articles were also retained at the entrance. (f) The checking also included removal of all packing material and wrappers from soaps, toothpaste and creams etc. These are specifically mentioned because these were noticed as articles used in bartering for the addicting substances. Sh. Satpal performed his duties most vigilantly and perfectly.

8. The Cook : Smt. Surjit Kaur was appointed as the cook in 2003 for the newly started kitchen for preparation of main meals, breakfast, and evening tea for the inmates. She also maintained the accounts of purchases and consumption in the kitchen. The addicts are generally very critical of the taste of the food served but the cook always managed to keep them satisfied and this made their stay more pleasant and the task of managing them in the Centre easier. The cleanliness of the kitchen and the hygienic perspectives were well attended by the cook.

9. The Yoga Therapist : Sh. Yash Kumar joined the Centre as a yoga therapist in the year 2002 and continued until the year 2010. Classes of physical Yoga were held every morning in the prayer room. He had a difficult duty of convincing the addicts about the benefits of physical yoga in their recovery. Being an experienced person in this field he managed very well and helped the addicts to share their personal problems related

to drug abuse and any personal problems not disclosed to the counsellor; his timely advice helped them to complete their treatment course.

10. The Safai Sewak: - There were number of changes of the persons appointed on this post. The duties of the *safai sewaks* were largely confined to the general cleanliness of the ward rooms and offices of the Centre with special emphasis on the cleanliness of the wards, the bathing rooms and the toilets.

STAFF MEMBERS AS TEAM WORKERS

The whole staff worked as a cohesive team attending to their respective duties efficiently, and all shared their daily observations on the addicts, with colleagues in the Centre. This provided daily information on all the activities of those under treatment and gave a broader perspective for improvement in the management. The Centre continued to grow in terms of a better understanding of the addicts, provision of facilities for the inmates and their response to treatment.

The Doctor, the Project in-Charge /Project Director, and the Nurse served in the Centre together for fifteen years from 1995 to early 2011. The ward boy, the gatekeeper, the cook and the yoga therapist, all appointed in 2002-2003, remained in service up to beginning of 2011. The long period of working and learning together was of great value towards a better understanding of "drug-addiction as a disease" and the addict its victim, as an individual.

The details with which the duties of each staff member have been described are meant to draw the attention of all concerned, to the various facets of "**The Disease Drug-addiction and its victim the addict** ", **and also how The Red Cross De-addiction-cum Rehabilitation Centre, Amritsar, was administered. All efforts were aimed at providing the best possible attention, care and environment, to encourage the addict to complete the course of indoor stay and move on to a satisfactory De-addicted status, Recovery and Rehabilitation.**

Appointment of a 'Pathi' in the Centre : The prayer meetings were held in the morning. This appointment was made very soon after the start of the Centre and continued for about a year. The addicts admitted for ten to fifteen days' indoor treatment were unable to benefit much because of the severe withdrawal physical discomfort in the first ten days. The 'Pathi ' stopped attending his duty and the post was abolished because of financial constraints mentioned earlier. The other staff members, especially the Experiential counsellors, motivated the inmates on the basis of self-experience, to spend time in the prayer room.

Computer Coach : Appointment of a computer coach Sh. Narinder Singh in the year 2008 was part of the plan to increase such services which helped 'the addict' to remain busy with some occupation and to disengage his thoughts from the addicting substances. The literate addicts appreciated this additional occupational therapy service and availed of this voluntarily. Sh. Narinder Singh was also a qualified electrician and trained the willing inmates in making minor electrical fittings.

ACCOMMODATION FACILITIES IN THE CENTRE:-

In 1995 the De-addiction Centre was expanded. The wards were shifted to the first floor of The Red Cross Sarai in Guru Nanak Dev Hospital Majitha Road, Amritsar. As the Centre developed further in its services and management, The Red Cross Office agreed to allow the use of the ground floor of the Sarai as well. The additional ground floor accommodation consisted of: (i) one main office room shared by the Project Co-ordinator/Project Director-cum-administrator and the visiting Doctor in-charge. In the same office, the Nurse prepared the daily prescriptions ordered by the Doctor. This was done directly under the supervision of the Project in-charge. (ii) Office cum counselling room for the counsellors with its door opening in the side corridor; all counselling session were held in it except the bed-side individual counselling when needed. (iii) Two wards with bed space for thirteen patients. (iv) Spacious dining room (v) **Prayer room.**(vi) A very long corridor in front of the rooms used by the patients for walk and exercise. The corridor was also used for viewing T.V. (vii) Six bathing cubicles and six toilet cubicles situated at the far end of the corridor.

The additional rooms on the ground floor included :- (a) **The office of the Project Director 'was the closest to the entrance door in the corridor'. This facilitated check of all those who entered the Centre, an additional safety measure against unwanted entries.** (b) The reception table in the side corridor adjacent to the main office, at the foot of the stairs; where the counsellor and the nurse received the addicts. (c) **The large prayer room was also used for physical yoga therapy, occupational therapy, family and inmates meetings and occasional visits of the school children brought by school authorities for awareness of addiction problem; the children were allowed to put questions to those under treatment.** (d) A spacious open space facing the corridor used for outdoor games such as basketball and badminton. The long corridor on the ground floor with double doors at the entrance, and bathing and toilet cubicles at the other end. (e) The wards for the patients were shifted to the first floor. One room on the ground floor was used for indoor games such as Table Tennis and the other was used as the dining room cum kitchenette. (f) The open courtyard on the ground floor opposite to the room for indoor games and the kitchen was surrounded by high walls. It was used for outdoor activities and games such as basketball. (g) A spacious kitchen for cooking, washing of the utensil and storage of ration.

Diet Schedule for the Inmates of the Centre:

Focus on nourishing diet was an important area of special care. In the beginning provision of food was arranged with a caterer and he supplied breakfast and the two main meals while the early morning tea and the evening tea was arranged by the Centre. **Some families offered to supplement the diet of their ward with milk, bread, fruit and even home-cooked food. This created problems of not only the entry of "addicting substances", but also of undesirable persons along with the food. This made checking at the entrance more cumbersome and ineffective in many cases. This system was also discontinued. Some families offered extra money**

for extra food facilities. **This was found not only problematic in account keeping but also in keeping the patients and the families satisfied.** Healthy, nourishing food prepared in the Centre, supplemented with a daily intake of Verka milk twice a day, curd, butter, and fresh fruit juice. The diet schedule given below was displayed near the entrance and the reception desk, for the patients and their families; with this display both the patients and the family could demand by right, if there was any lapse in the supply.

Diet Schedule

* Early morning tea.

*Breakfast: Stuffed paranthas with butter and a glass of milk. Bread was given to those who preferred it to paranthas.

*Mid-morning: A glass of fresh fruit juice.

*Lunch: Dal/vegetable/Black chana curry and chapattis and rice on demand. Fruit was given daily at lunch time.

*Evening tea: Tea with biscuits.

*Dinner: - Similar to the lunch menu alternating dal and vegetables as required.

*A glass of milk at bed time.

Over the years from 1995 to early 2011, the Centre improved steadily in its approach to giving the addicts best possible opportunities and environment helping them to move on towards effective De-addiction and Recovery. The essentials were: a) Medical treatment by the Doctor In-charge, a qualified psychiatrist. b) Proper care by the nurse and the other staff. c) Regular counselling of the individual addict and also with his family, and group counselling of the addicts. d) Nourishing diet. e) Comfortable stay. f) Complete sanitization against entry /availability of addicting substances. g) Occupational therapy sessions to minimize thoughts centred on the memory of 'drug - use' either individually or because of conversations / group discussion with other inmates.

FOLLOW-UP CARE / AFTER-CARE

The Ministry of Social Justice (M.S.J.E.) New Delhi recommends that the treated addicts should be provided follow-up care after discharge from a De-addiction Centre. This was ensured by The R.C.D.A.R.C. a) by follow-up visits of the treated addicts accompanied by the families. b) Home visits by the counsellors. These recommendations were followed by The R.C.D.A.R.C. Centre with some modifications as per utility and futility of these measures.

(A-i) Weekly/half monthly/monthly visits to the Centre:-The patients and the families co-operated; however, most of them continued to come for two/three / six months and some even up to one year. They were given counselling and medicines /tonics as needed. (A- ii) Follow-up visits and counselling sessions with Dr. Bhatia, the Doctor in-charge, at his clinic who put them on non-addicting substitute treatment, his treatment was complimentary. This follow- up scheme gave very good results in all the categories of addicts even in those who stayed for less than thirty days for Indoor treatment. **Unfortunately, a follow-up of this nature requiring repeated visits was acceptable to only a few families and still fewer addicts for obvious reasons.**

(B.) Telephonic follow-up: This proved to be the most effective programme. A fairly large number of the treated addicts could be followed for long period's upto two to three years and in few cases up to five years and even longer. The records of these visits were meticulously maintained by the Project Director herself.

(C.) **Follow-up home visits by the Counsellors :** This program was a failure in most cases due to lack of cooperation by the family; most of the time the addicts were not available at home at the time of visits. Parents did not co-operate and this programme was discontinued because of the above reason and also for non-productive financial burdens such as extra payment to the visiting counsellor and other related expenses.

(D.) **After – care in the Centre :** Of those who were willing to extend their stay in the Centre beyond one month in continuation of their indoor De-addiction treatment and whose families co-operated to pay for the extra period of indoor stay. These included: (1) Addicts who extended their In-house stay up to six months. (2) Those treated addicts who fulfilled the mandatory criteria of having remained drug-free for about a year and came as day time follow-up patients accompanied by their family and stayed during the working hours of the Centre. They remained under observation by the Project Director, the Doctor and The Counsellor. This plan proved an effective measure. Few of these were appointed counsellors and designated as Experimental Counsellors as recommended by M.S.J.E. New Delhi.

De-Addiction Supportive Services Provided by the Centre (listed earlier on page 97..... (Provison of services.... A) B) C)

Occupational Therapy :- During the indoor treatment, helping the addict to remain occupied and engrossed with some form of handwork, even if for one to two hours during the day, was very helpful. Such thought/mind engaging minor skills included:

a) Block printing: This was started soon after the Centre was opened; the printing blocks were made available by the R.C. Office. b) Painting of 'earthen deeva's and pots'; the counsellor Miss Prarthana actively participated in guiding the indoor patients. Deeva painting was discontinued in the subsequent year but the 'pot painting 'continued till the closure of the Centre as also the additional components of occupational therapy given below. c) Machine embroidery —initial training was given by a trained voluntary worker and later by an admitted addict trained by him, a professionalist in this art. Embroidery Machine was donated by a generous donor. d) Computer coaching — a qualified computer approach was appointed for this. **Of the two computers received as donation one was specifically for the coaching of the addicts under treatment. It was of great benefit to some of the addicts who showed keen interest in this activity.**

Prior to the appointment of the Computer coach in the Centre, the Experiential Counsellors (recovered addicts of The Centre) received computer training in the R.C. Office, Amritsar. Besides their contribution as Counsellors, they were an asset to the Centre in record maintenance and correspondence. Before the appointment of the computer coach they also trained the willing indoor addicts.

e) Making of electric switch boards— this became possible after the appointment of The Computer coach who was also a qualified electrician, a rare combination. Some addicts learnt with zeal; unfortunately, there is no follow up record.

f) Making decorative 'lurries 'of paper beadswere prepared from printed papers and those with floral designs and colourful background. The Project Director herself and the Counsellors trained the patients.

Indoor Games and Exercises on the ground floor

1. Basketball facility in the enclosed courtyard.
2. Table Tennis facility: This became possible after the Table for this game was donated by Sh. Raghunandan Bhatia. Honourable M .P. after his surprise visit to the Centre and his satisfaction with the management of the developing Centre. This activity proved an important contribution in motivating the addicts to prolong their stay and complete the course of their indoor treatment and even longer.

By the grace of God, the Centre continued, progressed, improved day by day and served more than two thousand seven hundred indoor addicts and their families in distress and nearly 7000 outdoor patients. Future ambitious plans for further improvement of the Centre remained

unrealised and came to a halt at the very beginning of the year 2011.

Specific features of the management of R.C.D.A.C / R.C.D.A.R.C Amritsar

Project in-charge, in a meeting with the whole staff, formulated a code of ethics to be observed while dealing with the addicts and also when interacting with their families. This was followed in letter and spirit. Short comings were corrected by interchange of information on the addicts under indoor treatment. All of us learnt to remain within the framework of these guidelines.

During the period of fifteen years that the Centre functioned, both Dr. J. P. S. Bhatia the Doctor in-charge and I as Project In-charge in various capacities worked together, overcoming all types of difficulties of red – tape restrictions. The objective was crystal clear — *The addict and his disease required adequate and appropriate treatment and holistic approach to management and taking bold constructive decisions undaunted and to the exclusion of all personal considerations. This was often misunderstood. However, we could continue to give our best, with the relentless service of the ward staff and the office staff and appreciative encouragement by the successive presidents and the chair persons of The Red Cross De-addiction-cum Rehabilitation Centre, Amritsar; any obstructive criticism from other quarters did not deter us.*

Inclusion of Drug- Addiction / Substance- Abuse, Alcohol Addiction as a Separate Subject in the Syllabus for Medical Under- Graduates in the M.B.B.S. Course

Drug-addiction is a disease and treatment of an addict requires an in-depth knowledge of what Drug-addiction/substance – abuse really means in terms of its effects on the body, mind and the personality of the addict and behavioural changes it causes in the addicted individual.

Drug/Substance abuse (drug addiction) is not mentioned amongst the diseases already included in the teaching curriculum of medical course; acceptance of Drug-addiction as a disease is relatively recent.

It is a disease about which the patient remains secretive, does not complain, does not seek medical attention and when brought to a De-addiction centre his denial is vehement and his cooperation is very poor for indoor admission and treatment.

Indoor treatment is an unavoidable essential step in the De-addiction regimes.

The De-addiction treatment regime consists of sequential phases during the De-addiction-cum-

Rehabilitation programmes. The awareness of this fact is very poor, both in the general public and even with most of the medical practitioners, who take up treatment of these patients sometimes by choice, or due to demanding circumstances because of the prevailing Drug-addiction scenario.

Many De-addiction Centres for indoor De-addiction treatment keep the patients for a pre-determined period of only ten to fifteen days. **This short period does not De-addict; such a short duration of indoor treatment Detoxifies, which is a mere preparatory stage and prepares him for the long-lasting Deaddiction regime that must follow. It is an essential key point in the treatment/management of Drug /substance-abuse victims.** The family of the Drug-addict has to be counselled on this point repeatedly, consistently and persistently and with tireless patience.

The standard Text Book of Pharmacology for teaching the undergraduates is*"Pharmacological Basis of Therapeutics* by Goodman and Gillman. It deals with the historical background and research papers pertaining to the addicting substances. These details are of academic value. There is incomplete information of practical management on the management of Drug-addiction as a disease. It does not prepare the medical graduate, the future practitioner for the practical difficulties that he is going to face in order appropriately to De - addict an addiction victim /substance-abuser.

The effect of addicting substances on the body and mind and the resultant behavioural and psychological changes, the occurrence of tolerance to addictive substance on repeated use, and the phenomena of withdrawal symptoms "The Abstinence Syndrome". All these are described in the existing contents of the approved curriculum. **The essential details for effectuating sustained and successful De-addiction, recovery and rehabilitation are not given.**

A Drug addict and his disease is perhaps the most challenging malady that has afflicted mankind and remains a medical dilemma up to date.

The Drug addict does not seek medical help on his own, rather avoids it. He denies being a Drug/substance - abuser, does not co-operate with the family, his response to counselling and advice is not steady, he can have wide mood swings even during the same day. The families of many addicts show a lack of co - operation; all this creates a problem in the handling of the difficulties during the treatment period. These and many other challenging situations are faced by those treating drug – addicts.

Each case of Drug addiction can disclose a new face of addiction/De-addiction problem. Each case requires an individual-specific and also a situation-specific approach. These and many other deductions have been drawn from my experience with more than 2700 indoor and over 7000 outpatients, during a span of fifteen years 1995-2010 / 11 in The Red Cross De-addiction –cum-Rehab. Centre (R.C.D.A.R.C) Amritsar, Punjab.

All the essential key points for successful and sustained / stable De-addiction cannot be learnt from books or conveyed through didactic teaching, however comprehensive it may be made. Drug – addiction / substance – abuse requires a specified

course on teaching on this disease, followed by supplementation with a training period for every medical graduate under an experienced De-addiction specialist.

The suggestion that the medical graduates should undergo a period of internship attachment and also post-graduation in the subject, merits serious consideration and early implementation for successfully managing a De-addiction cum Rehabilitation Centre.

The fact remains that the addicted population continues to rise both on account of new entrants as well as due to relapses in treated addicts believed to be successfully De-addicted. The failures are also due to inappropriate and inadequate management of Deaddiction regime, which itself is due to a lack of in-depth knowledge required insufficient details.

The need of the hour is a reappraisal of the existing efforts. So that every medical graduate is capable of dealing with the drug addiction/substance - abuse problem effectively. Therefore, the inclusion of treatment and management of drug-addicts / substance-abusers in the syllabus of medical undergraduates, specified period of internship and post-graduation in this subject merits an early consideration.

Addendum - 2

Co-relation of educational qualification, and the age of starting on 'DRUGS'. Data analysis of those admitted in The Red Cross De-addiction-cum-Rehabilitation Centre, Amritsar.

(Observations were made on the indoor patients of The Red Cross De-addiction-cum Rehabilitation Centre, Amritsar)

1.) **Educational qualification of those admitted for de-addiction treatment admitted from the year 2001-2010 — in terms of percentage of the yearly admission**

(A.) Illiterate/limited capacity to read and write — 4.0 %

(B.) Primary pass — 7.4 %

(C.) Middle pass (under-Matriculation) — 10.3 %

(D.) **Matriculates — 32.46%**

(E.) **Higher secondary and +2 — 35.0 %**

(F.) **Graduate/post-graduate — 38.8 %**

(G.) Diploma course/skill training/technical training — 3.9 %

(H.) Qualified professionals Doctor/lawyer and other — 0.41 %

The highest percentage were of Graduates / post-graduate 38.8% , Higher Secondary and +2 (35.2%), matriculates (32.46%), and combined (67.66%). The lowest percentage (0.41 %) was that of the

Professionals. The low percentage in this group suggest that the highly educated and professionals are capable of protecting themselves from the environmental influence of the addicted population. The other likely explanation is that they are financially sound and can manage drug-abuse expenses as well as other household expenses concurrently.

2.) STARTING AGE OF DRUG/SUBSTANCE – ABUSE FROM THE YEAR 2001 TO 2010.

(Age groups and incidence percentage of the admitted addicts)

Year	6 to14 yrs	15 to 19 year	20 to 25 years	26 to 30 yrs	30 to 60 yrs plus
2001	3.0%	38.8%	30.49%	18.80%	6.98%
2002	2.79%	26.75%	38.76%	10.97%	7.71%
2003	1.99%	32.89%	46.84%	11.29%	8.30%
2004	4.13%	28.22%	50.00%	9.65%	7.92%
2005	8.86%	33.23%	35.56%	12.50%	9.63%
2006	3.49%	34.99%	44.00%	7.50%	6.00%
2007	5.94%	30.94%	38.83%	14.35%	8.41%
2008	9.12%	33.33%	34.78%	15.58%	7.00%
2009	13.62%	30.49%	30.62%	12.54%	7.52%
2010	7.45%	31.6%	42.34%	12.22%	9.44%
Range	1.99-13.62%	26.75-38.8%	30.49-50.0%	7.5-18.88%	6.0-9.63%

In the present scenario of drug substance-abuse there is urgent need for highly focussed attention on the factors which are leading to the above drug-addiction scenario. How a six-year-old child became a victim of addiction (see column 1 of the above table) is thought provoking. This child was brought to The R.C.D.A.R.C Centre, Amritsar, by his grandfather for consultation and advice. The boy sniffed petrol from a small bottle hung like a necklace around his neck. This little boy answered all queries defiantly. He disclosed that he helped his elder brother in siphoning petrol from one family scooter to another. He experienced pleasure on sniffing and when unable to do so he became restless and felt a strong urge to repeat sniffing. The frequency of such sniffing bouts increased gradually. His bonding with the petrol sniffing increased to the extent that he put petrol in a small bottle and hung it around his neck hidden keeping it hidden under his shirt buttons. He carried this all day long including during school hours and sniffed it many times during the day because without sniffing he felt restless and became irritable. **This is a classical example of progressing substance abuse in a helpless small child.**

CORRELATION BETWEEN (1) EDUCATIONAL QUALIFICATION AND (2) AGE OF STARTING ON DRUG-ABUSE, OF THOSE ADMITTED FOR DE-ADDICTION TREATMENT. DATA ANALYSIS FROM THE YEAR 2001-2010

The first impact of the analysis of the record data is, that specialists, highly educated with post-graduate qualifications and those with technical training came for admission to R.C.D.A.R.C Amritsar in small numbers. The other categories with low admission numbers were the illiterate and those with primary education only. A somewhat higher incidence was of the middle pass and the under matric. The highest percentage was of Graduates / post-graduate 38.8% , Higher Secondary and +2 (35.2%), matriculates (32.46%), and combined (67.66%).

A plausible deduction from the pattern of a frequency distribution is that the highly educated were able to keep themselves free from drug-abuse. The illiterates and the poorly educated were also admitted in low numbers possibly because this category is less exposed to the peer pressure of addicted students in the school. **It must be added here that the scenario has drastically changed in the last few years.**

In this context, it is pertinent to conclude from the frequency distribution of the starting age of drug-addiction given above that (a) the highest percentage is of those in the age range of 16-22 years. (b) The lowest starting age recorded in this study was a child of eight years. It is further added that the tabulated data shows that each successive year there is increase in the number of addicts below the age of sixteen years.

The maximum percentage of the matriculates and higher secondary / +2 coincides with the maximum percentage of the starting age from 16 to 22 years. This indicates the vulnerability of the school-going children and falling prey to drug abuse. As at present, a large number of school-going children are known to be taking drugs. In the earlier years, the older school children were involved; possibly initiated to drug abuse by the addicts hovering outside the school premises or by those in their neighbourhood at home. Those addicted in this manner are now becoming the nuclei for initiating more addicts within the school premises. As a result of this, a large number of school-going children are getting addicted and the starting age has fallen to as low as 7 to 8 years. Further worrisome fallouts of the involvement of school children are, growing inaptitude, passing exams by unfair means, aggressive behaviour in the schools and discontinuing studies under peer pressure, after primary, middle, matriculation and +1 (many of these included in the category of +2).

CONCLUSION

The data analysis given above should make us sit up and take effective measures in controlling addiction in school children if the youth power is to be saved from further extinction.

In the current 'addiction menace scenario' the alarm bells are ringing aloud, the red light alert is there without flickering. It is high time that we do not merely notice and talk about this national problem. Meaningful and result-oriented means are urgently needed. It is imperative that this message reaches the teaching institutions also for active participation in controlling the spread of addiction menace in the schools. Urgent steps are needed before we lose much more than what have we already lost.